New Year, Same You –

A guide to health and happiness at the size you are

By Julie *"Fattymustrun"* **Creffield**

New Year, Same You –
A guide to health and happiness
at the size you are

Copyright: Julie Creffield
Published: 14th December 2015
Publisher: The Fat Girls Guide to Running

Thank you for respecting the hard work of this author. Find out more about the author and upcoming books at www.thefatgirlsguidetorunning.co.uk join her popular Facebook community at www.facebook.com/thefatgirlsguidetorunning or follow her on twitter @fattymustrun

For my daughter Rose,
in case she ever questions my love for her
and for my mum who's love I should never have questioned

Contents

Introduction

Do you remember as a child how long a whole year felt to pass? Waiting for Christmas to come round, or finally being able to move up to junior school? It seemed like whenever you were really looking forward to something the waiting just went on for an age, with every day moving at the speed of 80s dial up.

As an adult of course, the months and years just seem to whizz past at the speed of light, with barely the time to move our winter clothes out of the cupboard before autumn is back upon us again. If anything, most of us I am sure would like the option of a massive red stop button to pause things for a bit so we can draw breath and catch up. Or how about a gadget that lets us just slow down the pace down altogether to something a little more manageable? What the heck, let's go all out and get me a reverse setting so I can start all over, erasing all the embarrassing bits of my life.

I simply couldn't wait to grow up when I was a child. I thought childhood was totally over rated filled with huge periods of nothingness and then short moments of high drama that even the cast of Eastenders would be proud of. As a frustrated youngster, I longed to become an adult as soon as humanly possible, in the hope that one day people might actually listen to me for a change and at last I would be able to make my own decisions and not be told what to do anymore.

Who was I kidding?

So you would think like most kids that my birthday might be the most exciting day of the year back then? Well, in all honesty, I can barely remember the detail of my birthdays growing up. Besides, I suppose, my 5th birthday when I had a shared party with my best friend, Alison Lawrence (there is photographic evidence which proves it), and my 10th birthday, when I went to see 42nd street at the Theatre Royal Drury Lane, and remember eating Burger King for the first time.

I am sure my birthdays were always great fun and mum did her best to make them special; I just can't really recall many of them. For me, the more memorable time of the year was always, without a doubt, the 24-hour period, which spanned New Year's Eve through to New Year's Day.

The last day of the year was exciting because there was normally a family gathering of some sort to enjoy, with mum's Scottish side celebrating Hogmanay and the 31st December also coinciding with my sister Jennies' birthday. However, if I had to just choose just one day, then it would have to be the very first day of the New Year that would really win the crown…that was my MOST favouritist day by far. Because, whilst everyone else lounged around nursing hangovers, eating what remained of the Xmas grub and watching the latest Spielberg film to be released on terrestrial TV, I was up in my room eagerly making a start on my new diary for the year ahead thinking about how much more exciting this year would be compared to the last and what I would do differently.

From about age 6 or 7, I started the diary writing habit, probably after reading about Anne Frank, Adrian Mole or even Oscar Wilde (I was an avid reader with somewhat advanced taste and interest in books at that age), trying my hardest to write something each day. Unfortunately, I found the novelty wore off some time around February or March as I tired of writing the same boring old stuff or got annoyed with one of my siblings finding the damn thing (no matter how well I hid it) and taking the mickey out of what they found in it. I mean at 8 and a half years of age nothing remotely remarkable was happening in my life, and there's only so many ways you can describe the routine of getting up, arguing with your siblings and enduring a day at primary school…it seriously was like groundhog day! So sadly none of those early manuscripts made it into my adulthood.

When I was 13 though, we were asked to write an autobiography in English class, which was rather exciting, as I had recently acquired an old (and I mean OLD) typewriter. I convinced my mum to buy a new ribbon for it and I sat for days on end fingers covered in ink and Tippex as I penned my masterpiece, cleverly entitled "one of six", as I am one of six children, in case you were wondering. I still have the project in its plastic document cover in a box of old schoolwork somewhere. It's not the most riveting of reads, but what it does highlight is my desire to make sense of and document my life somehow...perhaps to somehow make my existence on this planet mean something. I was clearly destined to become a blogger it seemed, even if I didn't know it back then, but I had to hone my skills and find discipline in my writing first...besides blogging didn't really become a thing until at least the noughties, well not in my mind anyway.

So to cut a long and rather uneventful story short, there were various attempts of diary writing in my early years, and the odd pen pal exchange with my great uncle Les, otherwise known as the Fleet Street Scavenger after years of writing for the British press. He was a dear old man, the brother of my nan, who in many ways inspired me to write with his simple piece of advice delivered in the style of an old Hollywood actor, "If you want to become a writer my dear, you must write and write often." But the real turning point for me in my fledgling writing career came the year that East 17 hit the number 1 spot with "Stay another day" ahhh the memories.

It was Christmas day in 1995, and I was at the ripe old age of 15, where by your belief in Santa Claus is well and truly gone, but you still get excited by the thoughts of Xmas, even if you know you are neither going to get kissed under the mistletoe nor get the Casio stereo system you really had your heart set on... However I was quite easily pleased when it came to presents growing up, I'm still the same these days really, you can't go wrong with socks, books or stationery, seriously...and of course a selection pack if there's one going spare, you see that's how rock and roll I am.

This particular year, my mum had bought me THE coolest bit of stationary imaginable...a Filofax! Not just any old Filofax; (OK spoiler alert) it wasn't even a Filofax at all; it was a knock off version but branded in the latest fad of black and white photography, stocked in Woolworths and designed to capture the imagination of pocket money rich teenage girls. It even had a lock on it...which is of course encouraged secrecy and the pursuit of illicit deeds, right? Or had my mum already got a duplicate key cut and this was all a trick to infiltrate my teenage existence?

So as I sat there on New Years Day 1996, I stroked my new bit of kit, flicking through the different sections wondering what I would write in it...what adventures I would have over the next 12 months to fill those pristine A5 pages? What secret codes could I create? What things would I keep note of? I almost had a kiss this year, so now with the prospect of boys on the horizon if ever I had a reason to keep a diary it was now.

And I did.

I wrote something every day for a whole year, stashing it under my mattress each night for safekeeping's even if most of its contents were absolute tripe. Reading it back now (yes I still have it in my possession) I can't believe: A) how dull my life was; B) how much I read into situations when it comes to creatures of the opposite sex; and C) how much insight and self awareness I had about the fact I was different to all my peers, even at that relatively early stage of my life.

So why am I telling you lot all about my immature diary writing antics? What does this have in the slightest to do with you and your health goals for the next 12 months? Well, like Steven Hawking, and various other geniuses over the years, I believe I have an interesting theory about time in relation to dieting and the like, and my diary writing habit kind of supports this theory, although its possibly not as scientific or academically sound as theirs...go figure!

Wait for it....

I believe that when it comes to ideas around health and wellbeing too many of us (and when I say us I am mainly for the purpose of this book talking about overweight women) are either looking into the future, in a "when I am a bit smaller I will..." kind of way, or looking into the past with a "back when I was smaller" mentality. There is no middle ground...almost like there is a big fat void in terms of accepting the realities of where we actually are now. We rarely make adaptations to our daily life to make us feel better in the here and now. Instead, we usually do things we know are good for us as a result of the fear and preoccupation we all have of getting old, getting fat, or getting cancer.

I know I for one, have been responsible for this behaviour too over the years. Through this book, and the review of my past musings, I am going to attempt to show you there is a better way of thinking about time in relation to any health changes you want to make and besides putting pen to paper in a diary format is a much cheaper form of therapy in my eyes.

The other reason I wanted to start this book with some talk about my stop/start diary writing habits is because, when I look back at my life, I realise that some of the most poignant moments to date I have somehow managed to document. The whole of my 16th year captured moments like: my first boyfriend; my first proper job and going to college. Then there was the diary I kept when I went travelling for just over 5 weeks around South East Asia, tracking the highs and lows of travelling in developing countries with a sister who hates bugs and doesn't actually like roughing it. And then I guess the most significant of all my journals is the one I kept during my pregnancy and the first year of Rose, my daughter's life, something I will treasure for ever more.

So, why is it that I managed to write consistently at these times, but not so much during the less significant moments of my life? Were these periods of time that self-reflection was absolutely necessary to my survival? Or times where I felt the most learning would surface through my experiences subsequently being committed to paper? Or was it simply down to circumstance or luck?

There are many self help gurus (not that I am for a moment suggesting I am one of them) out there who recommend journaling as a tool for self-discovery and to aid recovery from or understanding of the trauma many of us experience in life. In this modern technology driven world, I guess blogging has become the equivalent outlet for our thoughts, which is perhaps why everyone and their dog (quite literally) have one now and why (some) bloggers are more influential than the mainstream press...although clearly I am not including myself in that...YET!!

It took me a while to make the connection really.

I didn't really cotton on to the benefits of blogging that early; I had never even read a blog before starting my own one (www.thefatgirlsguidetorunning.co.uk) in 2010, which is a bit short sighted I guess. But once I got into it, I found blogging via the Internet was a perfect outlet for me. Finally I had an audience to listen to the boring tales of my haphazard running antics. I often wonder where I would be with my health and happiness if I hadn't stumbled across that "how to start a blog" article after coming dead last in a 10K race. Would I even still be running? Because at the time my running was very sporadic, and I soon realised that if I didn't run I had nothing to write about.

Over the past 5 years, I have kept a pretty detailed record of my journey with weight loss, fitness, health and happiness... Perhaps then, it's no surprise that I am going to recommend to you, that for this next year, the only resolution you are permitted to make is to keep a journal throughout...but more about resolutions and about journal keeping later.

For now, I want to leave you with two key passages from my 1995 diary:

January 1st
Unsurprisingly I didn't wake up until gone eleven, but I stayed in bed until 2pm just listening to the kids and Lily (who stayed over for some reason last night) screaming and mucking about. I went downstairs just in time for dinner; Tom Thumb was on the TV. I had a whole heap of college work to finish but I couldn't be arsed to even started so instead I sat in my room listening to The Eternal CD Lisa lent me last night. I went back down later cos mum wanted us to play Scategories and Yatzee. A bit of an uneventful day really, hopefully life will get a bit more exciting once I am back at 6th form...why is my life so dry during the holidays...seriously I don't know how much more "family time" I can take. Roll on next week. Oh forgot to say I had a really strange dream about you know who last night...I wonder if I will see him again on Thursday at youth club.

December 31st
Surprisingly I didn't even feel sick this morning, which is a miracle considering I drunk two thunderbirds AND a bottle of K cider last night after work, just as well they put us all in cabs after the party, I wouldn't have fancied getting the bus home. I don't know if kissing Jimmy's friend was such a good idea last night you know what them lot can be like, but fuck it. It's Jennies birthday today so mum cooked a really nice dinner, and cracked open her bottle of Bacardi before we all headed off to Kims. I wonder when mum will actually let me have a drink? Its not like I'm a fucking child anymore. The party was actually quite funny, we all took the piss out of Geoffs belly, and I got away with drinking baileys when nobody was

watching. Oh well so technically speaking its actually 1996 now (I'm catching up on my diary a day after events). I wonder what this year will bring, cos this one has been pretty cool. I still haven't found love but I have had fun looking for it, and I now have some wicked friends...and me and mum are even getting on better now I am not with Jason anymore. I think I've learned a lot about where my priorities are and who my real friends actually are...plus I've stopped caring what other people think of me anyway. I don't know if I will make it as an actress, but I'm giving it a good go...just need to make sure I don't get kicked out of college again. 1995 had its highs and lows but all in all it's been a good year. This is Julie Creffield saying thank you diary for sharing all my experiences. If anyone reads this I hope you learn from it. Goodbye.

Yes I actually wrote all that shit!!!!

Please tell me my writing has a little more style and substance these days! But do you know what, in some ways it really doesn't matter. Diaries on the whole are not designed to be read by others, they are yours and yours alone...unless you are Oscar Wilde or Bridget Jones of course. Who cares if they are dull, or repetitive, or egotistical or self indulgent...because it's actually not even about the words on the page, it's about the process of collating your thoughts into something solid...turning your thoughts into real life things...words. Words that can be reread, re interpreted, rewritten at a later date even.

When I read back my diary from 1995 I am instantly transformed back to the 90s. I can remember exactly how I felt: the things which troubled me; what I was wearing; how I did my make up; what our home was like...despite the fact my writing wasn't very descriptive. I have an emotional connection to my experiences as I recall them, and in some ways reading them back acts as the most soothing forms of therapy.

The words remind me that I existed. I lived and I loved and despite not being perfectly formed as an adult or having all the answers, I still had something to say, meaning that it counts for something...if only to me. But hey, who else matters?

Task 1 – Buy yourself a journal

Visit your favourite stationers and buy the most luxurious or functional (whichever you prefer) notebook you can purchase for the sole purpose of keeping a journal. You can blog if you prefer but just know the process of other people reading your content may force you to over-think things and write what you think people want to hear.

Prepare yourself to start writing. This can be from this very moment, or you can wait until the 1st of January, whichever you prefer... However, a bit of advice: there is no time like the present. Later on in the book we are going to look at the reasons we procrastinate and prefer to start things on the first of something, be it a week, a month or a year...break the mould: do it your way instead.

Just start writing in this first instance whatever comes into your mind about the past year, your current state of physical and mental health and your hopes for the next 12 months. Over the consequent chapters, I will suggest specific topics or areas to focus on in your journaling, but remember there is no right or wrong way. If you really struggle to put pen to paper, try writing about some of the following...

- What you did today?
- How you feel about life?
- Your hopes for tomorrow?
- What you are concerned about?
- Who is impacting on your life and how

- Any external influences like quotes you come across, or world events

Do whatever feels right for you. Just don't procrastinate. Write in the morning, write before bed, write whenever you get the urge...just write.

How to approach this book

Women need real moments of solitude and self-reflection to balance out how much of ourselves we give away. **Barbara de Angelis, Writer**

Not that I am suggesting you are thick and don't know how to read a book, but speaking from my own experience, and I read hundreds of books each year (seriously), the ones which stick with me are the ones where I can apply the principles in a practical way, so please bear with me on this. You are taking the time to read it when you could be doing a million other things so the least I can do is make it easy for you. I really want you to get something quite specific from reading this particular book but as with anything, the more you put in the more you will get out of it.

You have probably downloaded and started to read this e-book sometime between December and February, not because this is the best time for self reflection or extreme lifestyle changes I might add, but because the whole premise of this book is about challenging the idea of New Year's Resolutions, especially health or weight loss related ones.

At this time of the year the media are bombarding us with January detox programmes, and how to lose the half stone you put on over Xmas articles, so its not the worst time to be armed with an alternative view on such matters. Besides, I worked my arse off in October and November to get this book finished so I would meet my publishing deadline, so please God, say at least a few of you did manage to get hold of it in time for 2016.

However, if you have downloaded this at any other time in the future there is no reason to not follow the instructions as they are laid out, as the points are valid all year round. Which will just go on to prove my theory even further, and I can promote the book throughout the year instead of just expecting a peak in sales over the winter period. Here's hoping!

But seriously, this book is designed to be read cover to cover, (hang on a second how does that even work for ebooks?) introducing a new but hopefully connected theme with each new chapter, alongside a number of coordinating tasks like Task One that suggests you start journaling.

The tasks are a mixture, of grab a piece of paper and write a list and think about this for a few moment tasks, and you can also write your thoughts on these specific areas in your journal as and when things become clear in your mind. Now of course it is completely up to you whether you attempt these tasks or not. I have simply included them to get you to engage a little deeper with the concepts of the book and to help you delve into some of the blockages you may have faced over the last few years. The journaling is key though so if you only do one thing make it be that...even if you burn the bloody thing afterwards.

I guess I should introduce myself to you, as its quite possible you are not one of my existing followers, who I initially had in my mind when writing this book...well I'd like to think it's being read by other women too.

My business card says, 'Julie Creffield Plus Size Athlete, Campaigner, Speaker and Author'...yep it really says all of those things; I never could decide to be just one thing and I guess it sounds better than Fat marathon runner who blogs about her experiences. Right?

I set up my blog The Fat Girls Guide to Running after coming dead last in a race in 2010. By the time I reached the finishing area, the finish line had been dismantled and everyone had gone home. I was incredibly embarrassed at the time, but later that night I saw the funny side of it and thought "this can't just happen to me" and did a quick Google search for "Fat women who run". There was very little information out there about running as a larger lady...there was a whole heap about running for weight loss though, the web was full of people trying to sell me something that would make me a slimmer, and therefore a better runner.

It took me less than 6 months to establish a following of my blog, which basically talked about the odd, frustrating and sometimes simply crazy things that happened to me while out running. So it was clear there was a gap in the market and there were other fat runners out there experiencing similar issues. A few years later, while on a bit of a break from working (yes I was unemployed and with a small baby to look after too), I realised that perhaps I should focus on the blog fulltime. I had just been told by my doctor that I was "Too Fat to Run" which outraged me and I started looking into the deep seeded problems overweight women face when it comes to making health changes.

I don't profess to be an academic expert on health, but I have spent the last 10 years or so fighting against the diet industry and the crap that comes with being an overweight woman in today's image obsessed world. Through my blog and the community of awesome women I have met along the way, I have had the luxury of being able to explore and challenge my own perceptions of what the pursuit of health should look like. Call it action research if you like. Although I am not able to report on any major weight loss personally in the last few months, recently I find myself in the happiest place of my life for a long time, despite going through a range of really stressful changes this year.

Perhaps I should have saved writing this book for when (or if ever) I lose a substantial amount of weight, or make my millions as an entrepreneur helping other women, but I don't buy into the whole before and after mindset we seem to be obsessed with. I simply feel compelled to share what I have learned so far whilst on this journey...NOW.

I already have 4 running related books on Amazon, and a 5th book in draft format all about how to improve speed…I just have to apply the principles myself and get my 5K time under 30 minutes (current PB 30.07). I knew I wanted to write a more general book on my story but in many ways I was waiting for some kind of conclusion to arrive in terms of my own health…because spoiler alert: I AM STILL FAT!!!! But do you know what? That's kind of the point. Health is not all about transformation, and I can (and do) still influence the lives of thousands of women around the world just as I am.

The idea for this specific book came to me last year when I purposely refrained from doing a big push on my online running club (www.toofattorun.co.uk/theclubhouse) during the January health and fitness rush, out of principle mostly, despite the reality that I probably lost revenue for my business by doing so. Why did I do it then? Because I refuse to be part of the diet and fitness industry and the media's obsession with fat shaming and wowing people with weight loss solutions for the 6 weeks immediately after the 1st January. All you need to do is look at the front pages of women's magazines during that time to see the kind of titles that just reek of propaganda…all those "lose 10lbs in 10days" and "detox your Xmas belly away." Headlines that make you feel crap about yourself at a time where you should be excited about the future.

Now I am all for being all motivated at the start of each New Year, and using it as a time for reflection of what has passed and the setting of new goals for the future, but trust me January is not the best time for setting health related resolutions, and I will explain why that is later in the book. I am just sick to death of the seasonal binge and restrict culture that has been created to help sell diet products, weight loss programmes and their accompanying goods and services each year, in a global industry worth an estimated 600 billion dollars, according to a report written by marketsandmarkets.com. It's clearly big business, but it doesn't mean it's right and that there is nothing we can each do about it.

This book is written with fat women in mind (although the messages are as valid for non fat women) so let me just share my take on this emotive word.

For as long as I care to remember I have always been called FAT, if ever someone was rude to me, or I argued with my siblings, friends or later on partners, whenever someone wanted to hurt me the F word would always surface. The times I sat in tears after complete strangers commented on my weight are too many to count. However a few years into writing my blog, I realised that the word no longer had that effect on me and I felt an enormous sense of relief. Many women who have bought my 'Too Fat to Run' merchandise tell me that by reclaiming the word they feel empowered in a way they didn't ever imagine possible. Now I know many women still feel very nervous about the use of the word, and it is still used to shame and blame overweight women, but I do think when you look at the word as a descriptor rather than an insult it helps take the power out of it. I will talk a little more about fat politics as a topic later.

Will this book help you lose weight? Who knows, only you can answer that, and it will depend on whether that is a true ambition of yours in the first place...I make no promises. What I can predict though, is that you will never see New Year in the same light again. You may even meet next year's midnight countdown feeling lighter than you ever have, if only from the lack of blame and shame about your current size and the lightness of mood which comes about when you begin to take your health and general wellbeing more seriously.

For me this eBook signifies a commitment from me to never to again buy into the ludicrous media foray that is January. I will not buy into the annual peddling of false hopes and I refuse to be part of the problem. This book is an attempt to get hundreds and thousands (perhaps even millions) of women to do the same, by becoming living breathing advocates for my Revolt Against Resolutions campaign. Or RAR as I like to call it.

Add a few As and Hs in between for effect if you like, and then get all animalistic and shout it out a few times, until you feel the right level of anger to drive you forward.

RaaaaaaaaaaaaaaaahhhhhhhhhRRRRRRR!!!!!

Ready for some action? Let's get started.

Task 2 – Declare your Revolt Against Hideous Resolutions
Tell the world that you are taking no further part in any of this New Year Resolution shite...and share the love by including the link to this book if you like.

Commit to becoming part of the solution rather than perpetuating the problem by explaining to people why living in the now is a much better idea than creating a resolution, which is destined to fail.

Don't listen with interest as people reel of their New Year Resolution lists, don't ask the question when you go back to work, and of course don't click on any links that buy into that methodology in any way shape or form.

Think about what you want to be; what you want to have; what you want to do...rather than what you don't. Then start actually doing it....even if we haven't yet got to the actual New Year yet.

Why resolutions REALLY don't work

I hope everyone that is reading this is having a really good day. And if you are not, just know that in every new minute that passes you have an opportunity to change that. **Gillian Anderson, Actress**

We've all been there haven't we? We feel our waistlines increasing (as they should by a few pounds) over the winter months as we move less and eat more comforting foods, and we think…ahhh sod it I'll wait for the New Year. I mean there's no point in starting anything now, Christmas is almost upon us…so we write off November and December, pinning our hopes on January 1st.

But of course we were out (or in) drinking and eating copious amounts of indulgent foods and drinks last night weren't we? Seeing in the New Year with a bang once more. So the following morning we are possibly feeling a little worse for wear…so porridge and green tea and a trip to the gym is never going to happen.

Plus, we still have a cupboard full of Xmas stuff, gifts, uneaten cheeses and boxes of cakes and sweets; oh and the Gym doesn't open until next week. Nope. We will wait till that lots all gone and then we will start properly with our new regime on Monday. So depending on where the Monday actually starts in the New Year, we could be on the 2nd, the 3rd or even the 6th. Hardly worth doing it at all now right 'cos I've blown it? Its not even a week into the New Year and you are already feeling like a looser.

OK so I am being pedantic

Plenty of people set New Year's Resolutions and keep them; otherwise the concept would have died out years ago? Right? Wrong! Research carried out by Scranton University in the United States showed that 40% of Americans made resolutions, yet only 8% of people stuck to them. The study found that for 2015 the top resolutions were,

1. Lose Weight
2. Get organised
3. Spend Less, Save more
4. Enjoy Life to the fullest
5. Staying or becoming fit and healthy
6. Learn something exciting
7. Quit Smoking
8. Help others in their dreams
9. Fall in love
10. Spend more time with family

And at least 6 of these have been frequent things on my resolution lists in the past, how about yours?

It's hardly surprising that weight loss is so high up on the priorities list seeing as global obesity has more than doubled since the 80s, which is ironic seeing as the 80s was when the aerobics and diet industries really seemed to ramp up their efforts. But how many of the other goals on that list have we put off in our pursuit of being slimmer, or equally are goals that go hand and hand with it?

So where did the habit of setting New Year's resolutions come from anyway? Good old Wikipedia says,

A **New Year's resolution** is a tradition, most common in the Western Hemisphere but also found in the Eastern Hemisphere, in which a person makes a promise to do an act of self-improvement or something slightly nice, such as opening doors for people beginning from New Year's Day.

I love the "slightly nice" bit, and I'd never heard it described in that way before. OK how about doing the world a favour and banishing the diet mentality? That would be nice. But how about stopping the blame and shame culture for women who don't fit what society deems as the norm full stop? Gee that would be pretty cool to attempt ever year wouldn't it?

And have you noticed that lots of New Year's resolutions tend to be about giving up so-called bad stuff? I'm giving up alcohol; I'm giving up chocolate; I'm gonna' stop biting my nails; I'm gonna' stop dating losers...Surely in a laws of attraction kind of way, with that mindset we are completely focussing on the negative, and therefore that is all the universe hears, making it of course more likely to happen. Because we all know now that what you think is what you become, right? Don't eat the chocolate, don't eat the chocolate...oh shit, I can't stop thinking about chocolate; sod it, I will have some chocolate.

It's like when you have small kids. You say, "Don't touch the vase, don't touch the vase." All the poor kid hears is "Vase" and before you know it they are obsessed with the damn thing and you know its only going to end up one way...broke.

Why are we so obsessed with what we don't want? We are anti war; against cruelty; fighting discrimination; we want to get rid of crime; eliminate child poverty; battle alcoholism and most importantly fight the fat - come on folks wake up! All that energy spent on the very things we don't want, and with resolutions they are often about giving things up or not doing the terrible things we have been doing of late.

A 2007 study by Richard Wiseman from the University of Bristol involving 3,000 people showed that 88% of those who set New Year's resolutions fail, despite the fact that 52% of the study's participants were confident of success at the beginning. Well, we are always positive at the start of a new regime, because the reality of the actual commitment is never properly thought through. Surprisingly, Men achieved their goal 22% more often when specific measurable goal targets were set. I guess because of their competitive nature, whereas women succeeded 10% more when they made their goals public and got support from their friends.

I don't buy into this whole SMART goal way of thinking anyway. I prefer to think of my goals as STUPID instead and I will explain why. Specific, Measurable, Achievable, Realistic and Timely can be left to the big boys of management consultancy because Walt Disney taught us if you can dream it your can achieve it without any talk of specificness. He also suggested that elephants might fly, which of course they do when being transported from one zoo to another; so it's all about perspective.

Back in 2005 when I set myself the goal of running a marathon, I weighed close to twenty stone. I had never run for more than 30 seconds straight, what was I thinking? My lifestyle was chaotic to say the least and I didn't have a great track record at sticking to things health and fitness related so running a full marathon was neither achievable nor realistic by anyone's standards...but I did manage it. I achieved that goal because I simply believed I could. I set myself targets, told others I would do it in the most public of ways and foolhardily moved through my plan to its competition...no matter what.

Finding balance, a concept we will explore in more detail later, has been my life's work and is something I still have to work hard on each and every day so that it doesn't slip away altogether. In the past I have often felt like the little girl with the little curl, no middle ground...either very very good or simply horrid, unfortunately both in my past behaviour and eating habits. I can be quite obsessive when it comes to getting something I really really want. Once I have set my heart on what I want I am unstoppable. Whether that is pulling the fittest boy at youth club as a teenager, or more appropriately getting my first class degree. Those massive challenges have all been eventually realised by having a huge goal, surrounded by an even huger desire to succeed, and a lust for achieving things that not everyone can get or do.

This is what I like to call having a BIG FAT STUPID Goal, similar in principle to Jim Collins' Big Hairy Audacious Goals. Goals that scare the living daylight out of you the moment you conceive them, making you feel slightly funny in your gut...leaving you with a "What if?" thought knocking about.

The difference is my BIG FAT STUPID goals are...well full of FAT, but not the nasty clog up your arteries, sit on your hips kind of fat but the good indulgent FATs that nutritionists are always banging on about. This FAT is good for you, great even, it's necessary, it's rich and creamy and succulent, like the tastiest Greek salad loaded with olives and feta cheese and smothered in good quality olive oil, or home made guacamole with home made wholemeal pitas calorie ridden but good for the heart and the soul.

Ok, so let's stop talking about food and get back to the goals thing, why STUPID goals? When writing this section of the book I asked my followers on Facebook if they used SMART goals at all to aid their training, and I was bombarded with numerous "are you joking" "If only" type of comments. One lady however said her goals tended to be STUPID rather than SMART,

S = Silly – when said out loud to myself or others
T = Talked – about on Facebook/Twitter and down the pub...lots
U = Unrealistic – even by my own standards
P = Posted late at night – often under the influence of wine
I = Idiotic – only a fool would believe I could do it
D = Dreams – as in "in my dreams"

Although sent to me in jest I am sure, I love this approach and have taken it on, as a bit of a Mantra "are my goals STUPID enough?" I often ask myself, often leading me to increasing them in scale. I am a firm believer that if you are not living life on the edge then you are taking up too much room, and I already take up a whole heap of room as it is, so trust me, I am half way there already.

Mae West said, "Better to be looked over than overlooked" and I remind myself of that almost daily, as I face my fears and go for my somewhat ambitious dreams. Because what I fear most is not losing, or even looking stupid, it's the fear of missing the opportunity to be better than what I am now all together, especially if that fear is caused simply by what others might think of me.

Who cares if your dreams sound silly? The idea of inserting toxins into your face or having fat extracted using a hoover is kind of foolish, yet millions of women do it each year, and why would I care what other people think anyway?

Talked about on Facebook? Why not? Facebook is a place where dreams are made of, a place where we can adapt our virtual persona and be who we want to be...I have 12,000 women listening to my ramblings via Facebook so don't knock it.

Social media is a great way of being accountable and staying motivated in fitness. I lose track of the number of times where a virtual friend has literally cyber kicked me out the door to get my run in for the day.

Posted late at night? Who am I to say when is the right time to formalise your goals? For many of us who live busy lives the evening is the only time we get to relax, and think and if it takes wine then so be it, good wine helps lubricate the mind in a similar way that good oil works on joints. Whatever works for you.

Mae West also said "He who hesitates is a damned fool." Her fool was in fact a man (go figure), but I am sure the principle is transferable, besides how many so-called idiots turn out to be geniuses in the end?

And finally the "in my dreams" bit, well yes that's kind of the point isn't it, so why the hell not? It's called pushing the boundaries.

So with this kind lady's permission I am sticking with STUPID goals, and so should you. Let others around you believe they are STUPID and then quietly and humbly get on with achieving them in spite of the disbelievers.

So how is this different from setting a resolution?

The word resolution comes from the Latin word Resolvere, which means re loosen and later in Middle English meant to solve, disintegrate or dissolve...so now we are getting somewhere.

Resolution means "A firm decision to do or not to do something", but often our resolve disappears as life gets in the way, especially when we are doing something because we feel we ought to and don't particularly believe we will do it anyway. When our sense of Why isn't that strong.

But see how motivated you get when you have a cause behind you fuelling your fire. That's what Big Fat Stupid Goals do, because they are your making and they are so incredibly ambitious and have the potential to be life changing that you simply have to do whatever it takes to achieve them.

When I think about how much time and energy I have wasted over the years on dieting, and unfocussed training due to not having a sufficiently sized goal in mind...what could I have done in its place? Learned a new language; invented a cure for cancer; become a renowned artist?

A few years ago, I visited the artist Henry Moore's studios and gardens in Essex. I had always loved his sculptures, especially Old Flo who resides in East London near me, and I had a wonderful day walking around the vast open spaces and various workshops taking it all in. What I was astounded with was the amount of work he did, and how much unfinished works exist too. For those who don't know Henry Moore was a prolific artist, who created many thousands (yes thousands) of sculptures, drawings, prints, textile and tapestry designs over a period of more than seventy years...He was a busy man. I later found this quote from him,

I think in terms of the day's resolutions, not the years'. **Henry Moore, Artist**

Do you think that might be the key to his artistic efficiency? Not wasting a single day? Refocusing continually instead of waiting? Henry Moore was clearly a man on a mission to leave his mark; he was thinking big.

So, what you would do if time and money was no object and you knew that whatever you chose you couldn't fail at? What would you do with your life?

Task 3 – Set yourself a BIG FAT STUPID GOAL for 2016

Without thinking about the reality of your personal situation, without any restrictions, what ifs or but how's, you need to think about the biggest stupidest most glorious goal you could possibly achieve. This is not the place to write, "To get down to a size 8 and marry David Beckham", because, believe it or not, there are happier, more fulfilling things to aim towards. I mean have you heard him talk? The point is you need to expand your mind and reconsider what potentially your biggest wildest health or fitness related goal could be, and that may require some research.

Think broadly about the kind of goals these could be, for example would it be to:

- Compete in a specific sport
- Visit a specific place in the world (which seems well out of your reach)
- Become a yoga instructor or a personal trainer
- Get a qualification in an alternative therapy
- Start a family

- Climb a mountain
- Swim an ocean
- Become a model
- Leave your job and start a business

For the purposes of this book, the goal should be one that is likely to have a transformative affect on your health and wellbeing, even if it is simply in terms of pursuing a lifelong goal, which will bring you happiness and fulfilment.

And trust me on this one, setting a specific weight loss goal doesn't work for this; if it did surely you would have reached this weight or dress size before now, and without my help. Loosing weight might be a side effect of the goal you are going to choose, but it shouldn't be the goal itself.

You are probably reading this and thinking, "She's suggesting I run a Marathon and I can barely run for twenty minutes without thinking I am going to die, so why on earth would I consider signing up to a 26.2 mile run any time soon?" The thing is, when you can't run for 30 seconds, I might as well suggest you run for 5 hours as opposed to an hour, as it makes very little difference. But your goal doesn't have to be running related; it could be about climbing a mountain, travelling the world, going scuba diving, having a baby. It could be anything you set your mind on...but just remember to think BIG.

Task 4 – Tell someone about your Big Fat Stupid Goal

I know it's a little scary to expose your dreams, especially when they are as crazy as yours, but saying them out loud to another human being, or to the world via your Facebook account is what will kick start a new form of accountability in your life. As I said before, do not worry about the how you are going to do it (we will come to that later), just be confident in the fact you are going to do it, one way or another. Start talking about it like it's a done deal already....because it can be.

The illusion of time

So we are barely a quarter of the way through this book and you have already committed to changing your life in a big way, that didn't take long at all did it? And if you haven't set your Big Fat Stupid Goal yet, reread the last chapter again and again until you do.

So now that you are on track, congratulate yourself for making the hardest step of all: committing to change. But now we need to start thinking about the realities of actually doing it. Dreams are great, but achieving them is what we are actually after, right? And we want to do it this year of course, because life is too short to be waiting around for a better time, the perfect time...because that simply doesn't exist.

Time is a funny old thing really. We watch it. We fret over it. We waste it. We enjoy it. We look forward to it. We moan about it. And many of us stupidly believe we can manage it somehow, and get more of it by being smart. We can't, not really...because it cannot be managed...it just is what it is making us all absolutely equal and able to compete fairly on this planet that we call earth. We each have 24 hours a day to play with, 24 short hours to fill with purpose or to waste away as we so please. A day is just a day, a week is just a week, a year is just a year...yet some of us are amazing at making each day count, and others waste years doing the same old shit and expecting a different outcome.

What has this got to do with the price of fish though? Well, so much of our health motivations in life revolve around time, especially when it come to diets, fitness and weigh loss. "I'll start again Monday" we insist, or "If only I could get back to my pre-baby weight", or "I'll work harder on tomorrow's run" we try to convince ourselves, and I have been guilty of this too.

I have often been accused by those around me of either looking back on my past, reminiscing about the time I could get away with wearing white jeans, when I was smaller than I ever thought I was but just didn't appreciate it, or else looking to the future and hoping that time will return again... OK so I don't really have a desire to ever wear white jeans, actually, FUCK IT, why don't I just find a pair of white Jeans in a size 20 and totally rock them....just for old time's sake.

Since becoming a blogger though, I have been forced to look at the picture that is my life. The life experiences that have created the person (or monster) than I am today, especially in terms of the dates and order that things happened in. Journalists are always asking me for a linear timeline explaining when I did stuff, and what effect that had on my body, especially my dress size or weight... They are never that particularly interested in my overall health or well-being though...strange that. Besides, how many of us have a "at first I weighed this and now I weight this, tada" story to tell? That is the bullshit unachievable dream that that diet companies peddle, and we all know that diets don't work and that transformational pictures don't always tell us the whole picture.

But what does?

Task 5 – Create a Health and Happiness Timeline

Sit down and create a document that illustrates your journey so far. Do this using yearly markers and measure things such as weight, dress size, happiness, but also make notes about what else was going on in your life. Where were you working; when did you have children; which boyfriends did you have? Pinpoint the moment where you felt most confident; mark where things changed; moments where you may have had depression, or felt lonely or vulnerable. You might want to draw pictures, or do it as a simple timeline, however you are going to find the information easiest to read. I find using a table format most useful, but do it however you prefer.

When I sat down and did this exercise I was amazed at what came out. It was in many ways the first time I had ever seen my whole life mapped out so honestly. Seriously, it was like therapy looking at the correlation between the things that were happening in my life and my weight at the time, but also how I felt about my body in relation to the people I had around me. It's all common sense stuff, but too often we don't join up all the dots, we don't take time in this way, or perhaps we are simply too scared to.

Remember ladies, to be able to understand where you are going in life, you seriously have to take stock and deal with where you have been. Yet more than that, you have to start living in the present because that is where the magic happens after all.

Not all of us can afford therapy to undo the hurt and despair we experienced growing up, or to finally get over the mean and spiteful comments we have dealt with over as adults. By simply laying it out and accepting your story as part of your journey it will really help you move forward and take away some of the blame that we often shoulder ourselves.

Considering I come from a working class background surrounded by an extended family of builders and nursery nurses, somehow even at quite an early stage of my life, I managed to develop somewhat of a spiritual understanding of the world. Now please don't confuse this with religion. I was brought up as a catholic and even went to a convent school, but let's just say I had too many unanswered questions and couldn't abide by the rules to be considered a "Good Catholic Girl" but I digress.

I think part of my deeper understanding of the world and thirst for knowledge came from the fact I read heaps as a child. I loved books so much so that one year I received a set of encyclopaedia's, my siblings rolled around laughing when I was over the moon. I loved learning about new people, new ways of life, different eras. Despite loving my family and being relatively happy with my lot, I also wanted something different and at times felt like I was destined for something quite different to those around me. It is why I think I started collecting quotes from quite an early age....and this was before the deluge of infographics and positive messages bounding around on social media. You would often find me highlighting passages in books, cutting things out of newspapers, or scribbling things into the back pages of my notebooks...to be summoned on a later date.

"Shoot for the moon. Even if you miss, you'll land among the stars." I can remember reading this one over and over again as I prepared for university, not knowing if I would be back home within a few weeks, tail between my legs. I figured even if I failed and couldn't hack it at Uni I could at least say I tried, and surely I would learn something. I had to have faith.

Spirituality, by my definition, is about having true faith, but also about searching for a deeper understanding of the world and continually looking at the bigger picture in an attempt to truly see what is around us. It's not necessarily accepting either science or religion as the guiding light, but rather accepting there is something in the middle, which is about nature, and energy and people; that evolution is somehow being the best version of you. That's probably the crappiest explanation of spirituality that you will have ever heard but there it is nevertheless. It is this interest in the unknown that has kept me hungry for knowledge; hungry for the answers to some of the huge challenges we are facing globally with obesity and inactivity.

So through my in-depth research (yeah right) for this book, I have been trying to really define my thoughts on how you find balance in health, and perhaps even a zen like state for being...as an alternative to the diet obsessed, stressing about food, must get to the gym attitude that follows so many of us around these days.

How many start again Mondays have you been through? How many times have you been like, "This is my year I can feel it, this is the year I am going to finally get healthy, get lean" and hold your hands up if you have ever muttered to yourself those dreaded words, "Oh well, what the heck I'll start again tomorrow?"

But what if tomorrow never comes? No, seriously what if you are not here to try again tomorrow? Remember there is only one certainty in this world and that is that we are all going to die. Now that's not me being morbid, and it sure as hell isn't an attempt to shame you into taking better care of your health, it is just a reality check. I wasted a good ten years of my life yoyo dieting, always starting again on Monday, promising myself that next year would be a better year...it never is. Not until you start looking at your life in the here and now, and start actually living for the moment.

In his book, 'The Power of Now' Eckhart Toole says we must end the delusion of time, we must get rid of this perpetual trap of being in flipping states of anticipation and then of memory.

"Time isn't precious at all, because it is an illusion. What you perceive as precious is not time but the one point that is out of time. The Now. That is precious indeed. The more you are focused on time – past and future – the more you miss the now, the most precious thing there is."

We will talk about food in much more detail later in the book, but if you think about the way you eat with this theory in mind perhaps there is a better way to think about time and change. Often when we lose control with our eating we wait until the following week (if we are on it) or sometimes even the following month to put things right. What if we just gave our self a moment and then refocused on eating in a more mindful way? Surely that would lead to more consistency rather than giving us permission to binge?

So much of our day, for example, can be taken up with the thinking about food, shopping for food, preparing food, fighting the urge to eat food…yet when we do actually eat, often we just whoof it down at speed without even tasting it. We rarely enjoy the feelings and tastes of the food we eat. Yet food is one of life's absolute pleasures and we simply don't get the pleasure we probably should get from it. Possibly, if we did this a bit more we would hear the signals our body is constantly giving out about hunger levels and even the types of food our bodies are craving and be more satisfied.

We have simply stopped listening to our bodies….but more of that later.

Task 6 – Listen to your body's signals

Spend a day completely tuned into your body's signals by keeping a log. Write down every half hour how you are feeling. What thoughts, emotions and physical sensations you can feel, like needing to pee, being thirsty, or having aches and pains and see if you actually react to them or simply ignore them.

Generally speaking, how often do we reflect on how we are feeling? For some of us it might be at the end of a long day, or it may be when something amazing happens and we consider how lucky we are. As described in the opening of this book, we often reflect on how our lives are going at the end of the year, or instead at the end of relationships, or at the end of a job or work contract, or occasionally when something life changing happens in our lives like a death or world event. On the whole, we evaluate when things are coming to an end, but rarely throughout.

But that's silly right? That's like driving straight into a storm even though all the signs are telling you to turn back and find another route? Or waiting until your next 3 month check up, to go and get that pain in your chest examined. Dumb. Don't wait.

Health and happiness improvements can be made by making tiny little adjustments over time. They don't need to be massive big shifts especially if they are unlikely to stay, and you don't have to wait for the start of a new year, new month, new week or even new day to make the change.

Task 7 – Take Positive Action

Spend a week of taking action to get away from negative habits. Don't wait until Monday to do it, do it now, this very second.

If that means tipping away your fizzy drink, or putting your half eaten chocolate bar in the dustbin do it. Keep your "how am I feeling" radar switched on all week and when you are feeling low, depressed, unhappy, unhealthy, unloved, out of control...do something immediately which is going to make you feel better. Now I know sometimes when you are in that fog of unhappiness or stress it can be hard to break away, so here are some ideas of things you could try.

1. Stop the action that is creating the negative feeling – This could be an argument, a binge, boredom, watching rubbish TV, drinking alcohol, sleeping too much.
2. Change your environment – leave the room, house, town etc.
3. Get outside – Fresh air always makes you feel better.
4. Be around people who make you feel great – sometimes our loved ones are the actual problem, so choose who you spend time with carefully. Children and animals can really lift your spirits.
5. Try something new – A new activity or place can keep your brain occupied.

6. Do something for you – have a nice bath, paint your nails, go for a massage, cook something nutritious.

Eliminate the things that give you instant relief but add to the wider problem. Things like eating high sugar or fatty foods, these give you instant highs but then comes the regret and guilt, and the physical impact on your body as it digests the foods, but more of this later. The same is true of alcohol, or recreational drugs...or hanging out with folks who you know don't really have your best interests at heart. Learn to be alone and build strength rather than being in company that make you feel like crap.

And the trick is to do all of this now, not tomorrow, not next week and definitely not next year as your next New Year's resolution. Because if you don't have the resolve to do it now, what makes you think you will have the resolve come January next year?

One thing I have noticed through my years of yoyo dieting and working with ladies who are often frustrated by their weight or body size is, that women are terrible for feeling like they are either on or off their diet or fitness regimes. The problem with having such an all or nothing approach, is this can sometimes mean that one small indiscretion or step off plan can often lead to a feeling of failure which is subsequently followed by a sense of giving up. Then a whole raft of sabotaging actions and the promise (somewhere in the middle of that mess) that you will get back on the wagon (again) come Monday. This is the frustrating and relentless nature of dieting that seriously does as much harm to your mental health as it does your physical health, because its all about extremes.

Task 8 – Act NOW

Stop being a 'Start Again on Monday' (SAM) person, and instead commit to becoming a 'Resuming Operations Now' (RON) kind of person, leaving the so-called "bad behaviour" behind without a second thought.

SAM thinking is New Year's Resolution thinking in action, RON thinking is about accepting yourself and finding balance, being accountable and pursuing a happier healthier version of you, right now, at whatever size you may be.

The phrase, 'there is no time like the present' is key to this, and despite being a really corny thing to say, the present really is a gift so how come we don't often see it in that way? The point is to constantly ask yourself, how am I feeling right now, this very moment, and if you are not feeling great ask yourself what could I do to make myself feel better, feel better this very moment?

What can I (yes you) do (which means take action) to make me (because I am most important in this scenario) feel better (because that is what the pursuit of health and happiness is about)

What can you do now, this very minute to make you feel happier or be healthier?

Finally, we can't have a chapter on time without talking about the concept of death, and no this is not the point where I shame you for all your bad habits and scare you into changing them through a fear of dying; there's enough of out there as it is. No. This section is more about making the most out of your life and ensuring you leave the planet with as few regrets as possible.

Claire Hudson, the owner of the website www.thoughtbrick.com a place for meditation, yoga and life discussion posted a blog on Lifehack called 20 things People Regret the Most Before they Die,

1. I wish I'd cared less about what other people think.
2. I wish I had accomplished more.
3. I wish I had told __ how I truly felt.
4. I wish I had stood up for myself more.
5. I wish I had followed my passion in life.

6. I wish our last conversation hadn't been an argument.
7. I wish I had let my children grow up to be who they wanted to be.
8. I wish I had lived more in the moment.
9. I wish I had worked less.
10. I wish I had travelled more.
11. I wish I had trusted my gut rather than listening to everyone else.
12. I wish I'd taken better care of myself.
13. I wish I'd taken more risks.
14. I wish I'd had more time.
15. I wish I hadn't worried so much.
16. I wish I'd appreciated ___ more.
17. I wish I'd spent more time with my family.
18. I wish I hadn't taken myself so seriously.
19. I wish I'd done more for other people.
20. I wish I could have felt happier.

You see, not a single mention of weight, or appearance, or what clothes you wore. Life is not about these things, its about the relationships we have the experiences we have, and knowing you have truly been yourself and done as much as you can to fulfil your potential as a human being. Well that's what I think anyway.

The phrase, "Live this day as if it was your last" is of course overused, but if you take a moment each and every day to consider this thought then perhaps it still remains one of the most crucial questions we can ask.

If I died tomorrow, I would regret not reconciling with a number of individuals from my past, not telling my family I love them enough, not being bold enough in my companies growth, and most of all not having more fun.... see all things that can be rectified. It's never too late.

Task 9 – This might be quite an emotional thing to do (an even a little morbid), but give it a go. Write an obituary for you. Think about what you want to be remembered for and who would be left behind, missing you.

Many of us are very guarded when it comes to thinking about our own mortality let alone talking about it, and its often something we put to the back of our minds because its just to difficult to comprehend. But we must. Because I believe that each and every one of us were put on this planet for a reason, and if we do not think about such things there is a great possibility that the process of evolution will simply not occur.

You are an important part of the jigsaw, you are a vital cog in the mechanics of this world but sometimes it's difficult to see just how key you are, and therefore you deserve to be taken seriously as a player.

So often, overweight women (well women of all shapes and sizes really) feel like they are not important to the world at large and it's hardly any wonder they have this view when you take into consideration the soundtrack of abuse, distaste and distain many of us live our lives in.

We must be more mindful ladies, that is the key...we need to keep these issues at the forefront of our mind, challenge them, ponder on them, debate them, find ways of coping, solutions to make things better. Because we are crucial to the survival of our species, never forget that.

Women who have been caught up in the frustrations of yo yo dieting and disordered eating may well feel powerless to change their past histories, playing it over and over again beating ourselves up for each failed attempt at weight loss.

We may feel we have no way of affecting the future...but the present and how you feel about what is going on in the here and now? Well that my dear...that is yours alone, yours to do as you wish and nobody can take that power away from you without you giving them permission to do so.

Use the power of now.

Choose year round love

You can't forgive without loving. And I don't mean sentimentality. I don't mean mush. I mean having enough courage to stand up and say, "I forgive. I'm finished with it" **Maya Angelou, Writer**

People often get confused about the concept of love, believing that it is simply something you feel, or else something that people feel about you. It is not. Love is a verb, it is a doing word, an action, something which you do or have done to you…and more importantly than that, it is something which you can 100% choose for yourself.

So let us start this chapter with a few questions about love. Are you in Love? Do you love yourself? Do you love who you are at this very point in time? What you stand for? What you have achieved and done so far in your life? And while we are at it do you love your body? And the way you look?

Task 10 – What do you love about you?

Write yourself a list of all the things you love about you. I don't want to know about the stuff you are not so keen on, just the bits about you that you absolutely adore.

Come on there must be something…think harder.

When I first wrote this list, I struggled a bit too, because as women, we are not supposed to like ourselves very much are we? Unless we are absolutely perfect in every way, a bit like Mary Poppins, but it would be rude to imply we had it all…because being vain would suggest we were not perfect at all, so there goes that theory.

Besides, we are bombarded by the media with the idea of what the perfect woman should be like. How she should behave. What she should have, be and do, and of course, how she should look. How can we compete with that on any kind of level? Furthermore, why should we have to?

Do you know there once was a time where I was absolutely perfect? You too. And despite the fact I can't often get my mum to admit to it these days, I know that the moment I was born in the summer of 1978 with the soundtrack of Grease Lightening playing somewhere in the background (it wasn't really). I was absolutely perfect and I was truly loved.

I know this because I too am a mum, and the love I feel for my daughter is incredible. I know it's supposed to be like that, and I am sure as she gets older and more troublesome (which I am assuming she's likely to) my love for her may feel different, as she challenges me, and does things I am not so proud of in the same way I did to my mother (yeah sorry about that mum). But the love will never disappear but it will, I am sure change in its intensity.

We all grow up understanding that our parents love us unconditionally (underneath it all), and when you have kids of your own you understand that this is of course a complex relationship. However what I wasn't prepared for, when I became a mum in 2013, was how much I would be loved by my child, and how that would make me feel.

When Rose was born she was placed on my chest, all screwed up and bloody with a mop of black hair, her tiny eyes fixed on mine and in a single moment I realised I was actually her mum (9 months of carrying her clearly wasn't enough time for me to get the message). In that moment, I realised that no matter what I did, no matter how much I screwed up, I would always be her mum and she would always love me. It's the way the world is supposed to be of course, but it doesn't stop it from feeling incredible though. As she approaches her 3rd birthday, no matter how much time I spend away from home, how many times I tell her, "no more sweets" or scream, "go to bed NOW" after the 10th time of getting out of bed, she still loves me. She looks at me simply with love and doesn't see my inadequacies, or the things that I beat myself up about; she basically thinks that I am perfect, because in her eyes - I am.

So why is it that, despite being sandwiched between two generations of females that love me, I still have difficulties loving myself fully?

Task 11 – Who loves you and what exactly do they love about you?

Of course self-love is important, and key to our health and happiness, but sometimes when we have been in a really dark place it's hard to feel positive and we struggle to love ourselves like we should. This is where considering how others see us can help. But please notice this exercise can evoke emotions that make us realise that those who should love us, don't always do so in the most positive ways.

Close your eyes and think about someone who you know loves you unconditionally, just as you are right now, who doesn't want you to change. See yourself through their eyes and try to feel what they feel about you. Think about the compliments you get, the times these people have verbalised their love for you, or acted in a way which makes it explicit how much they love you just as you are. Remember how that feels and know that this kind of love is a great place to visit when you are having wobbles with your own love of self.

Now I do like myself. I think I'm all right. In fact occasionally, especially when I've done something particularly amazing, I think I'm pretty awesome but do I out and out love myself? Well, not 100% of the time. No. Why is that? Is it because the process of growing up in this horrible old world beats that love out of us somehow? Perhaps it is the media's portrayal of the perfect woman that has us all feeling ridiculously imperfect and inadequate?

After losing nearly 4 stone in weight during Marathon training in 2012, I put almost 5 stone back on during the 9 months of my pregnancy, which was down to nothing more than lack of exercise and eating too much cake. So with a 3-month-old baby, no job to go back to, no clothes that fit me and days on end to fill, I found myself at an all time low in terms of my health and confidence. I knew I had to get back to my running if I wanted to take back control of my life. My blog had sat almost redundant for 8 months as I had nothing really to write about, and I had barely left the house without Rose in tow, so if nothing else running might give me some independence back, and I summoned up all the courage I had and returned to parkrun.

Let me tell you, returning to running after pregnancy is incredibly hard.

Physically it's like you are in a completely new and alien body, scared your insides might fall out for a start, and your legs and internal organs simply can't do what they used to do. So combine all of that with the psychological crap going on in your head about how you look and how useless you are at everything, oh and the absolute crisis of identity your also having, it's any wonder women go back to it at all.

So what did I do to ensure I didn't wimp out?

I signed up for another marathon of course and, for a bit of motivation (and something to do with all that time I had on my hands), I borrowed a copy of the extremely popular book, "Run Fat Bitch Run" by Ruth Field from my local library….FUCKING HELL…turns out this was the absolute last thing I needed in my life at that point. I have never EVER read a book that has made me shake with rage; at one point I seriously thought I might explode, or have a heart attack. I was so upset by what I was reading I had to keep putting the thing down and go and do something nice to calm down.

At first, I thought perhaps I was just a bit jealous that this other writer was having some success with a publication that sat in the market place I was writing in too? Nope. That was not it. I was just incredibly disappointed that a woman would want other women to feel so bloody crap about themselves, and that this book was so shamelessly being peddled to overweight women. It's been proven time and time again that shaming does nothing to motivate women to make changes, and here was all of of this unnecessary vileness coming from a woman who admits she had never actually been that overweight. Reviews on Amazon about this book were varied, with some women clearly responding well to the no nonsense tough love approach of the book, but this review summed up my views exactly making me realise that I was spot on with my analysis

So much of this book jarred with me. She encourages you to hate your body, to stand in front of the mirror (naked) and chant 'I'm a fat bitch'...why? Probably everyone who bought this book (for £10.99, mental) bought it because they are already unhappy with themselves - why make it worse? She then attempts to lighten the tone with 'oh, come on, it's just a laugh - I laugh at myself when I'm chanting this, it makes me megalolz, it's so funny ROFLcopter' but it's not funny, and it's not helpful.

I think it was the self-hate exercise with the mirror in the first few pages of the book that angered me most. So many women these days, overweight or otherwise, absolutely detest the way they look, or at least would prefer to look different if given the choice so the mirror is already a difficult enough place as it is to hang out in front of without the need to inflict a frequent barrage of abuse via it.

When I was at my largest, I didn't even own a mirror, and I avoided them in dressing rooms and the like too because my self-esteem was low enough as it was. I hated myself in photos, and became great at taking selfies in a way which disguised or cropped out altogether my growing body because I guess I was ashamed, and in denial about the extent of my disordered eating and inactive lifestyle. Plus I was too young back then to understand that my body was more than just the aesthetic casing that I lived in and in many ways I strongly believed I had a responsibility to be pleasing to the eye to those around me. What was that all about?

I guess I hadn't really thought about the real role my body played in the amazing story of my life, as my journey hadn't really begun. Years later though it became crystal clear. How can you hate your body when it has created life? How can you hate your body when it has successfully got you round 3 marathons and thousands of smaller races despite weighing what it does? Over the years my body has been through all sorts of traumas (some self inflicted and some not) and come out of it all reasonably unscathed. It houses me. It cradles my daughter when she is upset. It enables me to do and see amazing things without too many problems...why on earth should I hate or ignore it?

Task 12 – Ditch the diet books

Get any diet books or magazines you have knocking about which make you feel crap about yourself and destroy them symbolically or simply dispose of them, and don't ever buy any more again.

If you would like a recommendation for a book to fill the whopping big space on your bookshelf, there is one I might like to suggest. Louise Hay is the author of the bestselling book Heal Your Body which was published in 1976, two years before I was even born and long before it was at all fashionable to make the connection between the mind and body or write books about this.

She must have been able to predict the future because she has been saying for decades that as women we need to stop hating our bodies and instead choose love,

"I believe the best way to be good to your body is to remember to love it. Look into your own eyes in the mirror often. Tell yourself how wonderful you are. Give yourself a positive message every time you see your own reflection. Just love yourself. Don't wait until you become thin or build your muscles or lower your cholesterol or reduce your fat ratio. Just do it now"

If you have spent any number of years disliking your body, or even parts of your body, it can be difficult to change this mindset. We are encouraged to look at our bodies and see flaws and imperfections that are not there with terms such as problem areas, bingo wings, muffin tops and trouble spots. But what if you choose to love not hate the parts of your body that you have up until now spent so long hating?

Now I know what you might be thinking. You are probably looking at your belly, or your arms with feelings of loss, remembering how they once were and saying to yourself, "no amount of self love is going to change the fact my body now looks like this." I too have moments like this from time to time. But I have realised bombarding your body with messages of disgust does nothing other than bring you down and persuade you further to neglect or abuse your body.

I have always had "good legs", due to tap and ballet as a child, and then street dance as a teenager, and now running as an adult. So if I were to describe my legs to you, I would confidently say they are shapely, strong and attractive from ankle to mid thigh. I am not shy about getting them out on show, but my inner thighs (the bits that can't be seen when wearing a short dress) have a lot of area specific fat, and look just plain odd, which I used to be incredibly embarrassed of.

The area became a particular problem after my pregnancy, whereby I was losing the weight I had gained over the last 9 months equally from all the other areas of my body but the leg fat and loose skin, much to my annoyance, just remained...and I have hundreds of messages from women who say similar things about their bellies after having children.

It knocked my confidence, especially when my then partner suggested I did something to tone them up as I got undressed one night. His remark although he insists was not made to cause offence, hurt me incredibly and in some ways it motivated me to focus on that area even more in training. But let me tell you, no amount of squatting or inner thigh moves made a slight bit of difference, and I felt like I might as well give up.

This area of my body still looks about the same as it did two years ago, but I have learned firstly to accept this part of me rather than wishing it away. Consequently, I now make a point of looking at the area each and every day in a mirror but in a positive way rather than a negative way. I also take time to massage that part of my body, and apply moisturising cream daily too, as a reminder that this is apart of who I am and a part of my body that deserves to be cared for too.

Task 13 – Spend some time each and every day in front of the mirror.

Standing in front of a mirror and really looking at your own reflection takes some getting used to, but it is so important if you truly want to love your body and who you are as a person. Spending a few minutes every day to really see the whole you and not just a small selection of body parts you don't mind looking at will help you reconnect with your body.

If you don't feel to self conscious speak to your body, tell it why you love it so much and how much you appreciate what it does for you. Sending regular positive messages of love will make you feel so much better about yourself, even if you never lose a single pound ever again.

The greatest gifts you can give to yourself is not new clothes, or the most expensive make up (although these things have a place too), but it is self acceptance, self belief, self confidence and self love, and actually why stop at gifting just yourself with these things? Imagine what the world would be like if we shared these things with other females too.

I don't know if it's just me, but it seems these days that women are just absolutely obsessed with each other's bodies. Maybe it is the rise of reality TV, or Instagram or Celebrity culture. But even in the real world we compare, we contrast, we catch sneaky looks in changing rooms and spend hours upon hours looking in magazines at either airbrushed representations of women, or the dreaded red circles exposing the realities of cellulite, stretch marks, sweat patches or body hair.

I remember being at secondary school and there being a scale of attractive girls which would be voted on frequently, and seeing this was an all girls' school looking back that was just weird. In my twenties I would often scan the room to see if I was the biggest, or the ugliest...not that I had an ambition to be the prettiest, I simply wanted to fit in and not stick out. Plus I wanted to know where I stood in the pecking order, to reassure myself I wasn't the most unattractive....although often I felt I was, and sometimes I may well have been. But hang on a minute why is that even a thing? My purpose on this planet is not to simply be attractive; I am under no obligation to look good...so why do we have this crazy notion in our head?

At a social gathering I held at my home a few months ago, some old friends and I were talking about girls who went to our secondary school when someone said, "Oh my days, have you seen" such and such?" (I won't expose the poor girls name), and a number of the girls who were in this particular girls year at school knew exactly what she was referring too. This girl had got FAT all of a sudden. Now this was a particularly horrible, vain, self obsessed individual, who I remember clearly from school, but it was like these girls (my sister's friends in fact) were taking some comfort in the fact that this particular girl is apparently far from perfect these days, despite the fact that many of the group had experienced weight gain themselves. Like it was a curse, but somehow she deserved it.

I hold my hands up. I didn't challenge it at the time because I had a house full of guests and didn't want to ruin the night, but it's a feeling I have encountered a number of other times too. It's sometimes hard to challenge these kinds of conversations as they arise.

The level of fat shaming in real life, and increasingly on social media, is incredible, and often people don't even realise they are doing it. Over the years, I have caught many a celebrity (often males, I must add) taking the micky or sharing images in a way to shame women's bodies.

But even when we are not shaming the so-called 'non perfect bodies' we often hate on the 'perfect' ones too, with conversations like...

"Sarah's lost a whole heap of weight"
"Bitch"
"Well she's still got a big nose"
"I bet she thinks she's it right now"

If we can't love and appreciate women's bodies of all shapes and sizes and refrain from character judgements based purely on size or shape, what hope have we got for our own bodies?

Task 14a – Stop with the body hatred of other women.

For a week take note of how many judgements you make about other people's size, positive or negative. Not everyone who is slim is happy and not everyone who is large is unhappy. Think about where you got these views from, refrain from commenting on other women's bodies, even out of praise. Instead learn to send messages of love to all women's bodies, in preparation for the love you will send to your own.

Task 14b – Purposefully love other women's bodies

This task may feel a little strange at first and will take a whole heap of practising in order to find a way of doing this that doesn't feel odd for either you or the women themselves. The main focus is to think nice thoughts about ALL womens bodies, and not in a "ooohhh bad cellulite but nice boobs" kinda way, this is more about loving the body in its entirety.

Opportunities to love other women's bodies may be more frequent than you at first would imagine, but some ideas for this could include

- Talking positively about your female friends and family members bodies, and discouraging them from discussing the individual parts they like
- Giving a hug, being a little bit more tactile, offering a massage or a foot rub, bodily contact. This may need to be built up over time, but so many of us are devoid of human contact and some of us even fear that our bodies are so bad that nobody would want to touch them
- Planning group activities that involve joyous movement, but where the exercise is secondary to the fun and laughter that the experience brings.
- Treating your loved ones to foods which are going to truly bring joy, thinking creatively about this, and ensuring your efforts are not adding to their food overwhelm or create guilt, so if chocolates then a tiny box of exquisite ones, if a

meal out then somewhere new and has healthier options on the menu. Cheering someone up with a cheap bottle of plonk, a frozen pizza and a tub of crap ice cream is not true love surely?

We will talk a lot more about this in our section on habits, but there is no time like the present to start loving yourself properly and small gestures of self love applied daily can really help you shift a negative mindset.

Task 15 – Get into the habit of loving yourself with daily actions of love

Make sure that every day you take at least 10 minutes and do something nice for you. Take time to adore your body, take care of your environment and your belongings. A long bath, a pedicure or popping your favourite CD on the player while cooking dinner will remind you that you are an individual who deserves love, just like everyone else you care for. Get in the habit of doing things for yourself that make you feel loved, even if you have other people to love you also...sometimes they forget, and besides self love is the foundation of happiness

Finding Balance

Beauty is only skin deep. I think what's really important is finding balance of mind, body and spirit. **Jennifer Lopez, Singer**

I often wondered in years gone past about how my life might have played out if I wasn't so FAT, if I hadn't had this frustrating, annoying on-going problem with my weight. (Remember that is how I used to think about my size; now I don't ponder on such things). Would I have been more successful? Would I have found myself a husband, or started a family earlier? Ultimately, would I have been any happier?

Who bloody cares!

It's one of those pointless, stupid things we fill our heads with like, "what would you do if you won the lottery" type of foolishness. Wishing yourself slim almost as a way of keeping us stuck in that place where "slim" is good and "fat" is bad, yet waiting for a magic wand to miraculously get us there.

But the media keep telling us that Fat is bad, a whole heap of folk around me over the years have confirmed this commonly held belief too.

Whether it's the school nurse and their ever so unhelpful note home about a child's BMI; the well-meaning auntie that mentions you're the biggest out of your cousins at a family gathering or the idiot in his white van winding down his window to let you know he has noticed you're fatness, you know just in case you hadn't noticed it yourself. Aside from being intrusive and uncalled for, theses experiences build up a catalogue of evidence to back up the theory that weight loss is the only way to stop the abuse and live a happier more valid existence.

In many ways FAT is the last acceptable form of discrimination on this planet, yet the damage it does continues to be crippling for millions of women, leading often to low self esteem, disordered eating and just a general sadness and underlying anger.

Task 16 – Identify those moments of abuse

Make a list of all the times you can recall that someone has openly discriminated you (and others you know) as a result of your size, then think about if there was anything you could have done to…

a) Prevent them abusing you
b) Have responded in any different way
c) Feel any different about the incident

I remember when I was about 19 or 20 it was a hot summers day and I was out on a date at a nearby country pub with a boyfriend having an amazing time. We were sitting in the sun drinking cider and basically just minding our own business enjoying each other's company. I decided to go to the bar to get us a top up, and can recall feeling really happy as I walked towards the entrance of the pub with two empty pint glasses noticing a group of about 5 lads sitting on a bench nearby. That's when I heard one of them say (clearly loud enough for me to hear), "Oi Paul, here's one for ya, I know you like a big bird" to which of course they all laughed almost to the point of falling over.

I was stunned and walked into the bar as fast as I could, forgetting the drinks I had come into buy and instead running into the toilets to hide my tears. I sat in that cubicle for ages crying (and trying not to be heard) and basically feeling really crap about myself as a result of complete strangers and on what should have been a really happy day.

Despite that incident being close to twenty years ago, I will never forget just how powerless I felt at being unable to retaliate.

However, I have realised over the years that no response from me at all would ever have made them change their perspective, or their sense of entitlement to make women the butt of their jokes. Men (or should I say boys) like that will always exist, and I sure as hell didn't have the ability to challenge them in any useful way. Or at least I didn't think so.

This is just one example of being heckled or directly abused and, sadly, there are many more I could talk about. But the final straw came when an actual boyfriend called me a "Fat Bitch" in a heated row, which absolutely shocked me and cut me to the core. I realised in that moment that I had to do something about how I dealt with this kind of behaviour. Because as a larger than average person, it is clearly the most obvious tool for hurting you.

When I set up The Fat Girls Guide to Running I did it thinking that very few people would read it, so I didn't really think about the consequences of having such a provocative title, or brand as it would later become. But it struck a chord with other overweight women and it didn't cause the upset or controversy that I feared it might once it became more popular. In fact very few people have taken offence to the name, and if ever they have it has always been ultra slim women with no experience of being overweight that are worried it might offend overweight women.

Task 17 – What were your earliest memories of weight talk

Think about when your first become aware of body discrimination, or discussions about weight. When did you first start using the word fat as an insult (come on we have all done it) and were there other words you used to embarrass, hurt or annoy your friends or siblings? Can you remember how your parents would talk about putting on weight or the connection between weight and health?

Most of us learn that the word Fat is a naughty, insulting word from a really young age, and it's adults who often unknowingly teach us this, usually our parents or primary school teachers. The conversation usually goes a bit like this...

Child: Mummy Mummy, that man's FAT!!!! (said at the top of their voice)

Mum: (Clearly embarrassed) Shhhh, don't say that Brian

Child: Whhhyyyyyyyy?

Mum: Because it's not nice to call people FAT darling OK

Child: OK Mummy

And the child stores that information away for a later date, and remembers it when there are no adults around. "Ohhh I know a bad word, I know how I can get my sister back, I'll call her FAT"

Imagine if there was a completely different narrative to this? What if FAT was just a descriptor, what if it was the same as saying someone was tall, or blonde, or had freckles, you know a bit like the children's game "Who's Who?"

Player 1:   Does your person have red hair, no (Tap, Tap, Tap)

Player 2:   OK, is your person Fat (Yes) Tap, Tap, Tap, Tap

Player 1:   Is Mary your person???

Player 2:   Yep she is.

Player 1:   I win.

But how do you as a parent instil these kinds of beliefs in your children, when the world is telling them something else? Its not impossible, it just takes consistent considered reinforcement that people come in all shapes and sizes and that is fine. Then a conversation about a fat person might go like this instead,

Child: Mummy Mummy, that man's FAT!!!! (said at the top of their voice)

Mum: Yes, Brian he is isn't he.

Child: Like Auntie Julie

Mum: Yes that's right

Child: OK Mummy

And the child then thinks "ooohh I love Auntie Julie (I don't blame them 'cos she is pretty awesome), so Fat people are pretty much just like everyone else, just a bit more cuddly"

OK, so maybe that description is a bit simplistic but in an ideal word wouldn't we want all children growing up to accept diversity in all its forms, and simply be nice to everyone regardless of how they look?

The problem is there is still an underlying narrative that says overweight people are lazy, stupid, poor, a drain on resources and that as women especially we have a responsibility to be a certain size so that we are aesthetically pleasing to the eye.

It's all bullshit.

But is it secretly what we all want? Would we conform to the ideal body if we were given the choice? Sacrifice the amazing benefits of diversity and freedom to eat food in whichever way we choose and instead be a carbon copy of everyone else when it comes to body shape and diet choices for the foreseeable future?

Task 18 – What size would you like to be?

Without fear of judgement what do you think your ideal weight or size would be? How do you think your life would be different if you reached this goal? Is this target based on your experience of being this weight, or on a perception of what you think is appropriate?

I once went to this amazing health and fitness weekend with some friends that was unlike anything else I had ever been to. They are run by a company called 3Ness. They attract a different kind of crowd to the boot camps I had been on before and take a completely different approach with innovative new fitness crazes, high energy sessions with live DJs, and, get this, evening entertainment in the form of the hottest club nights...trust me they are great.

It was at this weekender that I met a weight loss coach that really made me think for the first time why it was I had never been successful in losing weight. Now he had an incredible story, he was severely overweight and had been most of his life. He showed a picture of him squeezed inside a bathtub, and he said he was extremely unhealthy and unhappy at a time where he should have been in his prime. He lost his weight through a well known diet (not one which I would endorse) and now he is one of their most successful licensed coaches or affiliates, whatever they are called, and I often have a nosy on his Facebook page to see the transformations he does with ladies, and it is mainly ladies.

But he told a story about when he had lost a few stone in the past, a number of his friends and family members started commenting saying "don't you think you have lost enough now", or would say things like "come on, have some pizza with us you've obviously got the weight thing under control now", like they were almost trying to ruin his efforts.

And this is a mindset we often find ourselves in. We go on a new regime, we change our lifestyles and we start to see the results, and then we plateau or find ourselves going back into our old behaviours and patterns, and often the people closest to us help us do it.

Is it self-sabotage? Is it because secretly we cannot deal with the reality of being a smaller version of ourselves? Are we scared of the power we have inside us to be amazing, and is it easier instead to yo yo between states, so we have something else (other than being the most phenomenal version of our self) to focus on?

Now I am not for a moment saying that you can only be happy, successful or at the top of your game when you are at what is considered a "normal" weight. However, I do think that most of us (when we are not yo-yoing) have a "natural weight"; a weight which suits our body structure and lifestyle best; where we feel comfortable and content; where we are not restricting our diets or exercising profusely to burn calories. But remember this natural weight will be different for each of us, and would still leave us in a world full of body diversity and would, I'm sure, include people who according to the medical profession would still be deemed overweight or obese.

So I guess the two big questions that I have had to think about for this book, but also in terms of the whole ethos and values of my company is,

1. **Can you ever truly love yourself if you still want to be smaller?**
2. **Is it OK to be an advocate for body positivity and diversity if you yourself want to change?**

Task 19 – What do you think about this?

Journalists ask me all the time, "what size would you like to be?" and I never know the answer, I never know if is a trick question and I am going to wake up to the tabloid headline of,

"Plus size body positivity campaigner secretly wants to be a size 12"

I can't ever remember a time where I was a size 12...it must have happened. I must just have missed it though because I feel like I have only ever been plus size (which isn't true as there are photos); yet I have difficulties picturing how I would feel or what impact this revelation would have on my life.

Being FAT is a big part of my identity. But equally I am asked often, "what are you going to do when you lose all your weight? You won't be able to represent the brand then hey?" For a while I thought these commentators had a point and was happily taking my eye off the ball nutrition wise (read stuffing my face), subconsciously rather than purposely, sabotaging my own health, in order to keep on brand.

Arrrgghhhh: the pressure.

And.

Do you know what?

I don't frigging well care what size I am, seriously.

I think I would be just as happy (or unhappy) at a size 12 as I am at a size 18 because what is important for me right now is my health and wellbeing. Although more importantly, I just want to find some bloody peace, some stability, some balance: I am sick and tired of being in a position of flux always seeking something else.

Now I have always been one for interesting words, but I hit the jackpot when at aged 16 I came across the following word,

Equilibrium

1.

A state of rest or balance due to the equal action of opposing forces.

2.Equal balance between any powers, influences, etc.; equality of effect.

3.Mental or emotional balance; equanimity

Or how I like to phrase it, Equilibrium- the natural state of balance.

Imagine waking up one day and not giving monkeys what you weigh today? Eating a delicious breakfast that sets you up for the day without any kind of dilemma over what to eat, or the guilty response afterwards. Picture fitting exercise into your day because you love it, rather than thinking you have to do it and having time in your day just to sit and be still and reflect on your life. Then finally, ending the day with thoughts of gratitude and a restful night's sleep.

Paradise hey?

I know that life can be challenging, and there are so many factors to consider in our lives these days, but surely balance (whatever this looks like for you) should be what we strive for.

Task 20a – What could balance look like for you?

Think about how you would feel if you found your natural weight and you never had to think about your weight again. If you had a lifestyle that involved balanced eating and joyful exercise that added value to your life. What words would you use to describe how you might feel?

Looking at those words, honestly ask yourself now, do I actually want to be slimmer or do I simply want to be happier? Is it really love and acceptance from the people I love and the world around me at large that I am seeking?

Task 20b – What would balance actually look like for you?

I want you to draw two pie charts, the first one splitting up roughly how you spend your time. This could be your average day in terms of hours, or it could be more how your priorities are split. So perhaps including things like, work, family, sleep, exercise, food, fun, friends. Now draw a second chart to indicate how a life of balance would look for you in an ideal world. What would you do more off, or less of? What would you get rid of all together or what might you introduce?

I have always been mindful of achieving a live work balance, I guess because I grew up with a mother who did everything for us and didn't really have much for her. When I first went into the work force, I worked hard and played hard and things seemed quite simple. Then as I got older, I found myself with more and more responsibilities and things to fill my time. Motherhood took this to a new level and I realised a few months ago that I can't do it all myself and that I would need to prioritise what was really important to me...hence the employment of a virtual assistant and a cleaner.

The point is so often we try to do everything our self, rarely asking for help... Even when it comes to dieting or making health changes, we believe we can do it alone or join well known dieting groups with regimes that take over our life, sucking the joy out of food and leaving us in a position where we feel powerless to keep it up without the structure of a programme.

Women over the past 50 years have been sucked into the diet mentality having been sold on the idea that being smaller will make you happier, and that it is just another thing to add to our list of things we must achieve in life. Surely we have missed the point completely? It is happiness that we should be seeking not a smaller backside or less cellulite. Just imagine what we could be getting on with in the world as women, if we were not wasting so much energy on dieting each year.

I bet mother Teresa didn't walk around complaining about her thighs, she had shit to do. Anonymous, Info graphic

In the next few chapters we are going to start talking about some specific behaviours and patterns that we sometimes fall into that have us stuck in a frustrating framework of being either good or bad, whether that's to do with food, or exercise or even our state of mental health and sleep patterns. This way of thinking is not helpful in any way, because what tends to follow is a sense of either entitlement and reward when you are "being good", or guilt and shame when you are "being bad", either way leading frequently to a string of disordered eating or blockages to do with self care and/or fitness.

The yoyo effect of being either 'on it' or 'off it' is confusing for your body, and is detrimental to your self esteem. Therefore we need to move away from this rhetoric and always think about health in terms of balance.

I like to think of it as a set of scales, not the ones you stand on but the old fashioned counterbalance weighing scales, where either side needs to have equal weight to be balanced. The next part of this book will show you what I think are the 6 fundamental ingredients which need to be represented, to some extent, on your health and happiness scale for true balance, and how you can avoid imbalances, even when individual elements of this simply cannot be achieved.

Finding your happy place where you feel in flow and control isn't easy, it takes honesty and hard work to make the adjustments that need to be made in your life. But trust me, the more mindful you can be of achieving balance the more likely you are to get there and life will become easier all round.

Remember it is near on impossible to be either be happy or healthy if your life is in free fall, and often it is the sense of being out of control, which is most damaging, rather than the behaviours themselves.

When you live in the now, purposely reviewing and adjusting your behaviour and not dwelling on anything for too long, you will feel more in control, namely because you have the tools to get yourself out of whatever funk you're in, be that food, exercise or mood.

When you live in the now, you manage how you think about yourself. You can tell yourself frequently that you are loved, and that you are enough as you are, and that you are living for the moment, but in the most positive of ways.

Habits of a lifetime

Times of transition are strenuous, but I love them. They are an opportunity to purge, rethink priorities, and be intentional about new habits. We can make our new normal any way we want. **Kristin Armstrong, Athlete**

Change is never as hard as you think it will be to make. Often it's the commitment to change that takes the longest, and the fear that surrounds that change which can lead to the most resistance.

I ummed and ahhed about joining a proper running club for almost 5 years. My running was no better when I eventually joined as it was four years previous, yet the fear I felt crippled me into inaction despite the fact I knew this one simple thing would transform my running. Once I had made the decision to actually do it: I felt like a weight had been lifted, and then all I had to do was turn up each week…and the improvements just came, as did an increase in confidence.

The best kind of change is the stuff that happens over time, because we know that massive lifestyle changes are quite difficult to maintain, especially if you don't have a good support network and a strong sense of WHY you are doing it in the first place.

In the last chapter I spoke about using the image of a balance scale as an indication of where you are currently at and for me there are 6 things that need to be represented on this counterbalance scale, which can easily be remembered as:

The three F's

1. Food
2. Fitness
3. Fun

And the three R's

1. Recovery
2. Rest
3. Relaxation

All six of these are key and I will go into much more detail about how you integrate this into your life without becoming a person you hardly recognise.

Task 21 – Score your level of balance

Take the lists above and give yourself a current score out of ten (1 being the lowest and 10 being the highest) for each of them. Try not to play the blame or shame game - this is not supposed to make you feel bad, it's just a baseline to show you where you are aligned and where you are not.

At this current time (as I sit here frantically trying to finish this book) my scores look a little like this

1. Food - 6
2. Fitness - 4
3. Fun - 4
4. Recovery - 5
5. Rest - 6
6. Relaxation – 5

These scores could be better, but what they do is let me know there is room for improvement. Also they help be to understand that the reason I am so tired and a little overwhelmed at present is because I am a little out of balance.

Given my current workload there are some things I have had to put on the backburner, like fun and fitness (which is at a bare minimum at present). Ensuring I get decent food and good quality sleep is what I have been focussing on to guarantee I don't have a meltdown of any sort….but it won't be like this forever.

This constant check and challenge is critical for me, as it should be for you.

You may look at me, or other fitness professionals or even friends of family members who manage to maintain a healthy lifestyle, and think, 'it's OK for you guys; this is your job; this is your life, or you have an advantage in some way'…I have a whole heap of other things on my plate to deal with too. I am a single mum, running a global business and bringing up a 3 year old on a budget so life isn't that straight forward for me either.

But even before I had kids, if I think about my lifestyle 10 or 15 years ago, it was just as manic, disorganised and usually involved me rushing from drama to drama. Basically, just about coping with the stresses and strains that life throws at you. Youth allows for that, luckily with very little impact on your health, but as you get older your body starts screaming at you to slow down and take better care of it, which is just as well really because otherwise we might never do so.

I never made all my changes in one fell swoop. I have basically carved out a lifestyle aligned to what I need right now based on habits, which I have picked up over time through trial and error, but as things change I will too. The point is I have started listening to my body and reflecting on what it, and my soul (which is quite important too), needs.

Task 22 - Identify and eliminate the blockages

For this task I would like you to draw a table. With the following headings in the columns:

- What are the biggest blockages to you leading a more healthier happier
- Who is responsible for these blockages
- Who contributed to them
- How might you unblock these
- Priorities (which are most pressing)
- When will you start

By putting your issues into some kind of priority list you can break down the scale of the problem into more manageable tasks so it doesn't feel so daunting. Often working on one issue or blockage will make the others simpler to tackle too.

Task 23 – Have a daily check in
Set an alarm on your phone to remind you to do a full health and happiness check each day. Think about how you are doing with 3 F's and 3 R's and perhaps give yourself a score out of ten as to how you think you are doing today.

You can combine this with your journal writing if that helps, or do it more as a 5 minute thought task somewhere in your day. Over time you can increase the number of times you check in with yourself, because each time you check in you are becoming more mindful and give yourself more and more opportunity to change your mood and reset yourself. This is a habit that I have created over the last six months which I have found invaluable, I call it my 3pm pit stop check.

Whenever I have worked in an office environment, I found myself always having a bit of a sugar dip come 3pm. I would feel drowsy, unmotivated, tired like I could lay under my desk and sleep, and usually just a bit cranky. I often took this as a cue to leave my desk, and often this was in pursuit of a chocolate bar or diet coke (urrghh don't ask).

As a stay at home mum and then a business owner working from home, I found that, despite the fact I didn't have the same working structure, I still had that 3pm dip. The difference is I was now either out and about and not taking much notice or it fell inline with a tea and coffee break, or else, when I was at home working, I'd take that as a cue to make a cupper, raid the biscuit tin, or if I was really shattered then have a nap.

The problem was I was feeling incredibly guilty about this gap in my day and making food choices that were not conducive to the way I wanted to eat. So I would start the day off really balanced, have a nutritious and delicious breakfast and lunch, but by 3pm I was stuffing my face with biscuits or cake knowing there were still a good few hours until dinner.

My therapist suggested that instead of trying to push past this down time I should encourage it and work with it. I am up at 7am every morning, and I often feel like I have done a days work before 9am just getting my daughter up and at nursery so my day can begin properly. On a typical busy day come 3pm, I have worked solidly for 8 hours it's no wonder I need a break. So what I do now is I have an alarm set on my activity tracker that buzzes on my wrist at 3pm and this instigates one of two responses.

1. If I am working from home I stop what I am doing and I think, 'am I hungry, am I thirsty or am I tired?' and I address each of those issues. I sometimes have a 45-minute sleep; I sometimes have a protein rich snack and then go and do some exercise like a brisk walk or swim; and sometimes I will simply have a cup of tea and a biscuit... Let me say that again...a biscuit and then come 4pm, I have an hour and a half left to play with until I have to pick up my daughter from nursery.

OR

2. If I am out of the office in the middle of something I take a few minutes to review how I am feeling. If I can I make my excuses then I pop off to the loo. If I can, I will find something healthy to eat, I will have a bit of a stretch, or I will pop into a café and have a hot drink and relax for a bit.

This is my thing. It has become my habit and I do it 95% of the time. It may not work for you, you may not need it, but it has transformed my life both in terms of my sense of wellbeing, but also in terms of my productivity.

You don't need to take any of my suggestions on board over the next few chapters, but what I would say is use the tasks ahead to try and identify what small things you could implement that would help you create healthier and happier habits.... Oh and try them out for at least a month before deciding if they work for you or not. The 3pm snooze thing felt counter intuitive at first, now I love my afternoon naps when I can get them.

Task 24 - Review old habits
What things have worked for you in the past that you could try again? What habits are you still doing that don't serve a purpose for you in your current life? What do people around you, who you admire, do religiously?

You will remember at the start of this book I asked you to keep a journal, not just because I enjoy writing but because I know it is one of those things that takes time and effort, and that sometimes the routine of doing it isn't that easy, but once you do it for a while it becomes a habit and one which comes with loads of benefits. So I hope you are getting into the habit of writing every day, if you haven't done so up until now, start today...diaries just like new habits don't need to be started at the beginning of the year.

When I was at university, I decided that at some point in my life I wanted to be a writer. My pen pal uncle Les who was a very successful writer would always say to me "If you want to be a writer you must write" and I was always frustrated with that response. I wanted him to tell me how exactly to do it. I wanted to get some insider knowledge or be given a foot up by getting some connections or something. But he never did that and my dream of being a writer was shelved. When my daughter was born the idea came to me again and I set about getting some stuff published. Within a few weeks I had 3 short articles in print, £250 in the bank and had started work on my first non-fiction book.

If you want to be a writer you have to write. If you want to be a runner you have to run. If you want to be healthier and happier...guess what you have to do? You just have to stop looking for the easy option and get on with the task every day. If you set about making small changes, incremental improvements, you will turn round one day and think "actually I am healthier and happier than what I was 6 months ago." But if you stick your head in the sand and do things like you always have done, moaning because you can't make all the big changes you'd like to, well sadly nothing much will change.

Task 25 – Undertake a workplace audit

(I was going to start this section off with a question about whether you work or not, but then realised just how stupid that sounds, all women work, whether they are in employment or not. What I do want you to do though is to review your working environment and think about the restrictions that are imposed as a result of the fact that so much of our time is dedicated to activities and tasks we have to do each week to make a living or keep a roof over our heads.)

Think about how active people are in your workplace. Is there a healthy culture or is it difficult to be more active or eat better in that environment. Think about where the health messaging is coming from (if at all), and what could easily be done to improve things?

The average person spends 50% of their waking day working. Let me say that again. Each day of your life that is a workday you will spend half of it at work. So that's a massive chunk of your life and depending on what kind of work you do has a massive impact on your health.

Office workers spend large parts of their day sitting on their backsides; night workers often get less daylight because they sleep during the day; similarly shift workers like nurses and doctors sleep at odd times and have varied patterns when it comes to eating and these work related habits have an impact on our health, and in many case our waist lines.

According to a Royal College of Physician's estimate, 700,000 NHS employees are obese, which is a little awkward when the NHS are key to providing services and messages around health and wellbeing to the general population.

Simon Stevens, the boss of NHS England has pleaded for all employers to do their bit to reduce the waistlines of the workforce and stop the NHS from sinking under the nations' weight, but in a Telegraph article last year the view was this was an embarrassing statement to make when the health service itself has some of the largest employees in the country. With the paper using phrases like, "Pot calling the kettle fat" and, "How can patients be expected to eat less and move more if those dishing out the advice are sitting down all day and picking at the Pringles" which I think is a bit harsh, and playing into the hands of the fat shaming blame culture which is prominent in the media.

Employers up and down the country though are being encouraged by the government to review the health and wellbeing provision for their staff, and it's in their interest to have a happy and healthy workforce, if for nothing more than staff retention, productivity and reduction in employee absenteeism.

Ultimately though, it is our responsibility to create good habits when it comes to our work. The trick is to work with your employers to create a culture where being active and eating well is the norm, and sometimes this requires workers to break the norm and challenge the status quo.

I once worked for a big public sector organisation that was very much a 'sit on you arse all day and eat cake that people had brought in' type, but over time I did see the culture change a bit. There were already showers in the basement, and bike storage so with a bit of encouragement from a few active souls it wasn't long before cycling to work wasn't seen as an odd thing to do, and lunch-time runs and yoga sessions were being held too.

Finally.

When it comes to habits, they sometimes take a while to embed, even with the best intentions in the world.

It is often misquoted that it takes just 21 days to form a habit. This snippet of sharable info came from a comment from plastic surgeon Dr Maltz who commented that it took his patients around 21 days to get used to their new nose or facelift, and even the consequences of having a limb removed. However, this observation has been twisted over time and used by a range of self help gurus and time management specialists to talk about how quickly you can shift from one way of thinking to another.

21 days is an OK amount of time to try out a new thing, but in my mind that amount of time still feels a bit gimmicky and could lead to real change not really being embedded, and old habits creeping back in once the "transformation" phase was over.

A more realistic timeframe I think is about 3 months, and this works well with the seasonality of the way we train. I always look at my training in 3-month blocks too, changing the theme or mindset of what I am doing to ensure I don't get bored.

Phillippa Lally is a health psychology researcher at University College London. In an article published in 2009 in the *European Journal of Social Psychology*, Lally and her research colleagues wanted to figure out how long it really takes to form a new habit.

The study looked at the habits of 96 people over a 12-week (3 month) period, with each participant choosing just one new habit for the duration and reporting each day on whether or not they did the behaviour and how automatic the behaviour felt.

For some this was a habit like "drinking a bottle of water with lunch." For others it was more difficult tasks like "running for 15 minutes before dinner." At the end of the 12 weeks, the researchers looked at the data to determine how long it took each person to go from starting a new behaviour to automatically doing it.

The answer?

The study concluded that on average, it takes more than 2 months before a new behaviour becomes automatic — 66 days to be exact. And how long it takes a new habit to form can vary widely depending on the behaviour, the person, and the circumstances.

In other words, if you want to set your expectations appropriately, the truth is that it will probably take you anywhere from two months to eight months to build a new behaviour into your life — not 21 days, so accepting that these changes are for the long term is your best bet and moving away from a quick fix mentality.

But what if you mess up and slip back into old habits, or a special occasion gets in the way? Interestingly, the researchers also found that "missing one opportunity to perform the behaviour did not materially affect the habit formation process." In other words, it doesn't matter if you mess up every now and then. Building better habits is not an all-or-nothing process.

But on the topic of special occasions, a few months ago I was lucky enough to see longevity specialist, keynote speaker and TV presenter, Tim Bean, give a talk on health and wellbeing whilst over from New Zealand on a short trip to London. I was thrilled to meet him over lunch and delighted that he knew who I was, "Ah you're the fat marathon runner lady who's all over social media" he said.

I really enjoyed his talk, but I must admit, I didn't agree with all of the techniques he described knowing that some of his messaging wouldn't work for me or my ladies, but remember he mainly works with men in male environments, often high achieving males, CEOs and the like, so it's not a huge problem that we have different approached. He did say one thing which really stuck with me when talking about food choices and the overwhelm we often feel,

"Its OK to have a treat on special occasions, but dinner is not a special occasion, dinner happens every fucking night"

He will probably hate me for quoting him on that, but it really resonated with me. If you are "treating" yourself with certain foods every bleeding day that becomes a habit, a habit that is going to be a huge struggle to drop, not only from a cravings point of view but also leave you with a feeling of a sense of loss or like you are being punished.

I know if you are an emotional eater (like me), or have tendencies of eating luxurious foods, because of a sense of entitlement; it is very easy to get into the habit of eating rich, calorie dense food every night. Having dessert and wine with dinner every night because you have had a hard day and you deserve a treat, a bit like being in holiday mode "go on, you're on holiday" comes the cry as you sit down for your third 3 course meal of the day.

We need to move away from this habit, and instead truly enjoy the treats when it is in fact a special occasion. Although in the UK I feel like so much is celebrated using food; it's like almost weekly, if not daily that it is someone's birthday at work, or a seasonal holiday where food based treats are the norm. My suggestion is to pick and choose which of these you want to celebrate and then politely reframe from participating in the others. Although, trust me, I know this is difficult and requires a lot of determination.

Food planning can be really helpful with this, particularly during times of the year where you know it's going to be difficult to maintain your healthier habits. I also find planning what I am going to eat leads to less waste and less stress about what to buy, what your going to cook, and whether you are getting a balanced diet – but more about that in our chapter on food.

Benjamin Franklin was spot on when he said, "by failing to prepare, you are preparing to fail." In the early days, when you are still forming your new habits, it is vital that you plan all 6 of my suggested elements of health and happiness so you can see where you are heading.

I find it a lot easier to plan and create new food and fitness habits. However, mindset or rest and relaxation ones require me to plan, schedule and diarise so they don't slip off my agenda when life gets busy.

Planning can also help you eliminate bad and unproductive habits like too much drinking or watching of crap TV, sometimes in tandem. So now rather than plonking myself in front of the TV at 6pm and realising at 10.30pm I haven't moved, I schedule which TV shows I want to watch, and I turn the TV off in between. My TV consumption on the whole lasts for 7-8 hours a week, and possibly the odd film...some people watch that much TV on a daily basis and then moan about not having enough time to workout.

In the past I have had messages from women I know asking for my help to get them fit and lose weight, I have always tried to help and will work with them to help them believe they can do it, because I want to help. Sometimes though these women don't really want to change and before you know it they message me saying they have too much on at the moment, and will get back to me in the New Year to join one of my online challenges... It doesn't take long for me then to notice their Facebook update about the goings on in terms of who's slagging off who on TOWIE or what's going down on Eastenders.

There is nothing wrong with television or any other activity to enjoy. Although sometimes you have to ask yourself if you are truly getting enjoyment from this activity or is it a habit that you have found yourself in which could be switched for something else that better serves you in the longer term?

"I find television very interesting. Every time somebody turns on the set, I go into the other room and read a book." **Groucho Marx**

Food

Eating well gives a spectacular joy to life and contributes immensely to goodwill and happy companionship. **Elsa Schiaparelli, Designer**

It has taken me the longest of times to understand, overstand and truly accept that my long-standing relationship with food is a key factor of both my initial weight gain in my late teens, and the subsequent trouble I have had losing that weight since.

If exercise alone made you thin...well, I'd be thin already right? Abs are made in the kitchen not the gym goes the fitspiration quote after all. Anyway we all know what we should eat really for a healthier life don't we? Well do we? Hmmmm???

January is the absolute worst time of year for adverts and marketing drives to get us all dieting (again) or eating healthy (whatever that may mean). So brace yourself for Weightwatchers and Slimming World Adverts and coupons in the papers, and no doubt all the supermarkets will be doing offers on chemically enhanced "healthy foods" and maybe even some fruit and veg to get us all in the 5 a day spirit.

I get panicky even thinking about it, and might even go cold turkey with my TV consumption during this time just to avoid it. I guess the food overwhelm is year round though, and for someone who has been on as many diets and food plans as me you get to the point where you simply don't trust your own judgement on anything anymore when it comes to food choices.

I believe we have reached a peak of absolute food overwhelm and deep ingrained hypocrisy when it comes to the messages around health that we are fed by the media and the powers that be. If red and processed meat is so bad for you, how come NHS hospitals still serve it to patients?

Over the past few years, I have found myself sitting on a Sunday night painfully planning out my meals for the week and literally having palpitations at the thought of having to go food shopping, not knowing what the hell I should be eating. Have you ever found yourself walking aimlessly round and round the supermarket with an empty trolley passing aisle after aisle of highly processed cleverly packaged food like products with their sneaky marketing, and their tempting buy one get 2 free offers at a loss for what to pick up for dinner? It's enough to drive a person insane.

Carbs? No carbs? Low carbs? Low sugar? Low fat? Good fat? Raw food? Liquid food? Convenience food? Superfood? Super value? Frozen? Fresh, tinned or vacuum packed? Fresh fruit, dried fruit or no fruit? Paleo? On the go? Low GI? High fibre? Vegan? Vegetarian? Gluten free? Dairy free? UUUURRRRGGGGHHHH! STOP ALREADY!

I first became aware of the link between what I ate and my weight at the age of about 12 or 13, as I watched my mum making up these weird looking pink shakes from a tin, in a similar way to how she made up my younger siblings baby formula neither looking very tasty. Of course I joined her a few years later on SlimFast too, as a way to control my teenage weight gain after a misplaced comment from a well meaning auntie who commented that I was getting "big". Weightwatchers came next and I had 4 or 5 bouts at that over a 15 year period. Then came the following of various diet books, Atkins, Low GI Diet, Dukan, Paleo...I was always looking for the next best thing, the thing which would finally help me shift my weight.

When I ask the women in my online running club about their experiences, many of them mirror mine, with so many of us having spent 20 years or more of our lives yoyo dieting, restricting food intake for a while followed by periods of binge eating, often turning to the foods we know deep down were not doing us any favours when it came to our health. Perhaps we were all feeding a completely different kind of hunger? But nobody really talks about this kind of addiction, and that is what it often is. I can admit it is only in the last 6 months or so that I have found the courage to say I have addictive behaviours around food, and that I need support in this area.

We all know that diets don't work. It's been documented time and time again with the initial weight loss often followed shortly by the weight piling back on again and more besides, with a narrative of, "well, I'm simply not disciplined enough" or, "what is wrong with me?" and the deep ingrained guilt and despair that comes with such apparent and often recurrent failure.

I can tell you, the simplistic message that comes from health professionals and naturally thin people of move more and eat less just does not ring true for women like me that have spent decades confusing their bodies with a constant barrage of hap hazard dietary campaigns. If only it was as simple as that.

Women tell me all the time that they just don't know what to do in terms of nutrition, they are at their wits end because there is so much conflicting information out there. "Just please tell me what to eat" comes the plea time and time again. But I am not an expert, and advice I give on eating only comes from my understanding of fuelling myself, and what works for me.

Part of the problem is we simply do not believe the experts any more, because everyone is selling you a dream...a dream that never seems to materialise which is why there has been a huge rise in healthy food bloggers with many of us preferring to put our trust in other every day women who are living with the same issues, even if these figures don't have letters after their name or a diet book to sell.

But who can we really trust?

Task 26 – Think about what food messages you were fed both as a child, and also the messages you now believe now you are more in control of your own food choices. Are they interconnected? Where did you learn about nutrition? Has it been influenced by diet programmes or systems? Who do you trust to give you sound nutritional advice? Are your eating habits still influenced by other people around you?

At the beginning of this year, I was asked to appear on Sky News Breakfast to discuss a new diet app coming onto the market. It was described to me as being similar to tinder, swipe right if a food is good for you and swipe left if its not. How simplistic? But is that really where we are going wrong? Now I am not a nutritionist and have no formal qualifications in this area, but I do feel like I have learned a little bit about how food works in the body, particularly in terms of fuelling me as an athlete, and I have basically just worked out what works for me...and isn't that the point.

That being said it doesn't mean I always follow my own advice, because food for me is still very much connected to my emotions, dealing with crap from my past oh and of course coping with the challenges that life throws at me.

Task 27 - Without reading the remainder of this chapter, use a blank piece of paper and compile two lists of foods that you know to be either good or bad, include the foods you tend to eat frequently, plus the ones you specifically avoid.

I guess I've never really had the healthiest relationship with food. For as long as I can remember, I have always been in an environment of feast and famine, whereby the cupboards and fridge were completely bare of overflowing with goodies. Growing up in a family with 6 children, you had to get in fast to get your share before some other bugger pinched it, and it was always about who had more chips than everyone else.

Food was always used as a treat, buttery toast after swimming, sweets with our pocket money, and chips and candyfloss whenever we went to the beach. I am not for a minute saying we grew up eating junk all of the time, Mum was a great cook and could make a mean roast dinner or lamb curry depending on her mood. But I did grow up in the 80s, which of course marked the height of convenience food, (oh and aerobics Jayne Fonda style) and I guess as a single parent of 6 growing kids cheap and readily available convenience food occasionally had its perks.

At 13 I got my first part time job working at my local Wimpy. That didn't really help with my growing waistline but this was more about gaining independence than it was about having access to unlimited food. My 12 hour shift would in fact entitle me to just two meals, but of course the choice was limited and there wasn't a salad to be found on that menu...so over the space of a weekend I would pack away 4 portions of burgers and chips, and as much fizzy pop as I fancied between serving customers.

Despite my early connection to fast food, I actually loved healthy foods as a child, and was never a vegetable dodger or a picky eater of any sort. I always thought that salads and fresh foods were what posh people ate, and I liked the feeling of eating above my station. I have always preferred what I consider "proper food", meals that are prepared from scratch over and above fast or convenient foods. My problem though, has always been about using food as a way of coping with life.

In the past, when I have been stressed, when I am particularly busy, when I am feeling upset, and sometimes even simply excited because something amazing has just happened, I tended to turn to food as my immediate response, and of course it's never a salad I reach out for. It's always high sugar, high salt or high fat content food...and quite often washed down with alcohol, which all come with their own unique hangover and guilt.

I think generally though we are too obsessed with whether food is good or bad. We tend to be either on or off our diet and our mood and how we view our self seems to be so closely linked to that premise. But let me tell you ladies, food is neither good or bad morally, you are not going to go straight to Hell simply because you like melted cheese on your burgers, but the diet and food industry will seriously have you believe that.

Just look at the crazy nature of how food is packaged and sold to us. We've all seen those "death by chocolate" products, and we do it our self too, with people describing their weekend fry ups as "a heart attack on a plate". And then on the opposite end of the scale the so called health products are marketed as being heavenly, or virtuous or guilt free, with images of nature, or children and even angels (chemically enhanced dessert and yogurt products in particular) used to reel us in and make us feel like we are being good for a change.

It has taken me a long time to realise that food is just food, and just as importantly for me, I now acknowledge it isn't going anywhere...if I buy a packet of biscuits I don't have to eat them all in one go, because none of my siblings are going to come along and eat them all before I get a look in, and even if they do I have the funds now to go and buy more if I want to.

The thing is I don't even particularly like biscuits....not that biscuits are bad, in fact there is an awesome little video on YouTube which illustrates this perfectly (you really should check this out)

But even if you are with me on the whole not labelling food as good and bad thing, I still think we have a responsibility to ourselves to think carefully about what we put in our bodies most of the time. Because food does, of course, have a nutritional value and can influence our physical, psychological and spiritual sense of wellbeing, and the more you can read up from reliable sources about the impact that foods have on the body and mind the better.

The past 12 months have been an absolute revolution and for me now, I don't touch diet products and I don't count calories or fat content. I don't avoid whole food groups (apart from gluten which I will talk about later), and I don't stress out about eating food I'd rather not as a result of eating out, or being somewhere where my preferred choices were not available. But most importantly, I have learned to listen to the signals my body clearly wants to give to me around fuelling myself.

There are 5 things I do now that stop me from falling back into a diet mindset, some of which are typical intuitive eating techniques or found in hypnotherapy programmes such as Paul McKenna's "I Can make you thin" book....but of course for me this is not about thinness this is about balance and feeling less out of control when it comes to food.

1. **I try only to eat when I am physically hungry** – If I find myself craving foods when I know I am not hungry, I ask myself what is going on. Am I thirsty, am I upset, am I stressed, or am I tired? Often the feeling passes, I grab an apple or I change my environment to avoid using food as a crutch. I also eat after 9pm, or outside meal times if I feel physically hungry...knowing that I am listening to the needs of my body

2. **I stop eating when I am full** – I eat slower these days and I try not to eat while doing other things, this stops me from missing the signal that tells me I am in fact full. What this often means is I am left with food on my plate, which is fine. I sometimes put this in a dish back in the fridge and sometimes I throw it away. It's only food and there is plenty more where it came from.

3. **I only eat foods I truly enjoy eating** – and this means I am experimenting more with cooking and trying new food

combinations when out an about, rather than sticking to things I habitually choose, which were often linked to being the lower calorie option or what is seen as forbidden. I say to myself, 'what do I REALLY want to eat?' And that is what I choose.

4. **I work hard to not be influenced by others** – I say no to food I don't want, without saying, "I am on a diet" or "I'm not allowed" by simply explaining I am not hungry, or I just don't fancy it. I also care less about what other people think when it comes to my food choices. If I fancy a burger I will have one, or I will order a salad if that's what I want, even when everyone else is enjoying pizza because that is fine too. I also don't mind being the social outcast at an event by bringing my own food, if that is what I have decided to do that day. It's my body and I get to decide what goes into it.

5. **I think of myself as an athlete** – I adjust my food intake according to what I feel my body needs to train at its best. I am aware of food groups such as protein, carbs and fat because I understand (enough) about the biomechanics of my body and what it needs to function, especially when my training increases or changes. I listen to my hunger as a guide and try not to use food as a reward for exercise.

That's all well and good I hear you say, but you still want to know what to actually eat? Or more importantly what not to? But as I explained earlier, I don't know you personally so how can I possibly try to influence your food choices?

I have been on a difficult twenty year journey of self discovery when it comes to food, and in many ways I know I've got a long way still to go on this issue. Despite not having cracked it fully myself, I have come to my own conclusions around things which seem to have worked for me in terms of balance, but only you can decide if this way of eating would work for you.

My diet at the moment tends to include proteins such as chicken, beef, fish and eggs, with a bit of dairy thrown in occasionally, and lots and lots of vegetables especially courgettes, sweet potatoes and butter nut squash which help bulk up meals and a bit of fruit here and there. In terms of carbs, I tend to stick with potatoes and brown rice, but also enjoy cous cous and quinoa occasionally too. I don't each much bread or pasta simply because it doesn't make me feel that great, however on a recent trip to Rome I had the best ever spaghetti and a scrummy pizza…but only because it was what I really wanted to eat.

I do eat other foods besides what I listed above, but I find I feel I have the most energy and am the most interested in food and cooking when I use the ingredients above. I must add though, I love using herbs and spices so what may look like a boring palette of foods to choose from, my love of Caribbean, Asian, Mediterranean and Middle Eastern cuisine means I am never bored.

It has taken me well over 20 years to learn enough about certain foods and how my body responds to them to be able to sensibly monitor my intake of these, and below I have listed 5 types of foods or drinks which although I enjoy sometimes, I am ultra aware of the consequences for me of over indulging in them.

- **Sugar** – I don't particularly have a sweet tooth. However I find, if I have access to lots of sweet food, I tend to over indulge in these just because they are there or because I crave them when feeling low. In the past, I used chocolate for example as a crutch at around 3pm when my blood sugars were low. Now I simply have a protein-based snack instead, meaning I don't have a crash an hour later, leaving me satisfied until dinnertime. I am also ultra aware of all the recent research into the addictive nature of sugar and sugar alternatives, and I find, personally, that the less of it I consume, the less of it I desire, meaning that I can enjoy the occasional slice of really delicious cake without the sense of guilt or the fear of overdoing it. I find it frightening the amount of added sugars in drinks and savoury foods, which is one of the reasons, I tend not to rely on processed or pre packaged foods; although sometimes I resort to these if there isn't an alternative.

- **Fat** – Butter, or marge, saturated or non-saturated? Urrrghhh, it's all a bit confusing right? Especially if you have lived through the Fat is bad years like I have, always choosing no or low fat options as a matter of habit. Well no more. Our bodies need fat and I make sure I get plenty of it in terms of variety. Olive oil, coconut oil, oily fish, nuts & seeds is where I get most of my fats and occasionally fat from dairy. A lot of processed foods have high levels of the bad fats that lead to high cholesterol and high blood pressure. You would be silly to ignore the information that is out there about the impact of high fat diets but this is about balance and common sense.

- **Carbs** – Carbohydrates get a bad press, and there are lots of low carb no carb diets which often claim huge weight loss results. But one of the problems with low carb diets is that you have no energy to do anything, which pretty much leaves you faint most of the time and unable to exercise properly. Carb intake should be reflective of how active you are and should be a compliment to your meal, not the main event. Eating refined carbs leads to sugar imbalances, for me, and overeating, in terms of portion control, so I am more mindful of this than any other area of my diet.

- **Alcohol** – I love myself an alcoholic drink or two. And although I don't drink as much or as frequently as I did in my twenties and early thirties, I still enjoy alcohol on special occasions and occasionally at other times. The difference is now I understand the consequences of drinking, which, for me, is: dealing with hangovers with a small child in my life; losing sight of my ideal food choices during and after my drinking; and the impact it has on my ability to train. Thankfully, my bingeing behaviour is a thing of the past though, because I know that, for me, drinking too much was always about being in a bad place and not having other ways to de-stress or switch off.

- **Fizzy Drinks** – I have always struggled with giving up diet drinks. Years of doing Weightwatchers ingrained the idea that a can of diet coke was an OK snack to see me between meals, or an alternative to having something else sweet that I was craving. I still drink the occasional can, and sometimes as a mixer with alcohol, but I don't use it as a crutch like I used to and again I now know the health implications that come with drinking fizzy drinks and make the choice consciously instead of unconsciously.

This has been the most difficult chapter for me to write in this book, for a similar reason as to why I don't write much about food and nutrition on my blog. I am not a qualified nutritionist or dietician, and I feel like a fraud giving advice on what to eat, when I haven't got this completely sussed myself. I think at the back of my mind I am also incredibly fearful about having what I say on this subject scrutinised and contested by other experts out there. I can almost hear them saying "And you wonder why you are still fat?" or "Well I simply don't believe you!"

There are so many contradictions at play when I think about my views on food and it has taken me a long time to accept that I have, for the past 20 years or so, suffered from disordered eating. No not an eating disorder. Disordered eating, because if I had a specific eating disorder I could get help, and people would understand my plight and perhaps have a bit more empathy. No, instead I have hidden my binge and restrict patterns of eating away, embarrassed that I simply have no self-control when it comes to food.

It's funny because I don't particularly have an addictive personality. I tried smoking at 14, didn't like it so didn't stick at it. I have had periods of heavy drinking (but often bingeing rather than addictive regular drinking). On addition, I even dabbled in recreational drugs after finishing university. However, I always managed to get my real highs elsewhere in life from work and other pursuits, and if ever I felt an inkling that I had a problem I was always able to stop.

With wider acknowledged addictions like alcoholism, drug abuse or gambling even, I often think it is an easier task to tackle (I know that sounds quite flippant). With support, or rehab etc. you can then just go cold turkey and avoid those things once you are clean. The problem with food is it is impossible to not eat, and wherever you are food is always there: you can't avoid it. Plus disordered eating isn't recognised as a real problem, instead you are just thought of as greedy, or glutinous or you have no self control.

Over the past few months, I have been working with a therapist to better understand my challenges with food. I have been tracking my food intake some weeks and sharing this with my personal trainer and I have realised that so many of my specific behaviours are not about food at all, but are about self worth, fears around poverty and being stuck in my past. Now that I am aware of my issues, it's a lot easier to acknowledge them and respond to them in a more positive way.

Even while writing this book, I noticed a specific behaviour that I needed to address. When I got tired from being at my desk for long periods I would make a cup of tea and grab an Eat Nature Bar, which is a great snack for me. It's gluten free, made of fruit and nuts and this particular one has dark chocolate on it too. It feels indulgent, but I know it has goodness within it too. The problem was, I found myself eating two of these with every cup of tea, and this disordered eating was not about hunger, it was about dealing with my stress. Once I noticed this, I said out loud to myself "Julie you have had one already and you really enjoyed it; one was plenty, and there are more in the cupboard if you truly want one later on."

It is not just overweight, or severely underweight people that have disordered eating. How many of us have eaten something until it has made us feel sick? Lots of us do that as kids, and some of us never grow out of it. How many of us find ourselves eating food that we don't even enjoy just because it is there, or finishing off a meal because someone has made it or paid for it although you are full up or don't really like the taste of it. It is OK to stop eating half way through; just tell yourself, 'I am not enjoying this, therefore I am going to stop'.

I am generally in a much better place now when it comes to what I put in my mouth, but I also know that this balancing act is a difficult one like with any addiction.

Task 28 – What food choices do you make for other people?

When you provide food for other people what set of thinking do you go through? Do you limit your kids' sugar intake? Do you avoid food with nuts in for Sue from across the road? Are you happy to go meat free for your stroppy teenage niece? Do you stop Uncle Bob drinking whisky because you know he has a problem with his liver? Of course you do. Because that is what responsible, caring friends and relatives do.

The process of weaning my daughter was like having an epiphany. Why would I not give her certain foods but happily stuff them down my throat? Just like I never got the whole "chicken nugget and chips for the kids and then steak in mushroom sauce for the adults" thing; nor the parents who prepare organic home made baby food for their toddler and thy are living on a diet of McDonalds and Cream Cakes.

Let me be explicit here. If weight loss is something you want and you are serious about pursuing this avenue - then you seriously need to be honest about your diet and seek professional help from a dietician or nutritionist to help create a bespoke plan that supports your training and lifestyle. This is not the same as going on a diet and while you still have this mindset nothing will change. Diets do not work. Therefore, I am not for a minute suggesting you need to diet, but this is about lifestyle change and, I know this is often a phrase used to describe diets, but no other phrase says what I want it to say... this is for life with the occasional allowance for moments of madness.

*Perseverance is failing 19 times and succeeding the 20th. **Julie Andrews***

Task 29 – Keep a 7-day food diary

This is a task you will often be asked to do when you are on a diet, or in fact when any health professional is giving you dietary advice. There are pros and cons to keeping food diaries, but I would suggest you keep one for the next 7 days so you can respond to this task and make your own mind up

The Pros – Being mindful of what goes in your mouth can be an eye opener, especially if you write absolutely every mouth full, and details on the brands and portions sizes you are using. If you know someone else may look at your diary this may help you avoid temptation, or think about whether you are getting the right balance of nutrients and food groups.

The Cons – It can become quite obsessive, you can start second guessing yourself and restricting your food intake even when you are physically hungry. It's tempting to lie, or miss out snacks etc. Sometimes the enjoyment of food is lacking when you are thinking about it all the time. The pressure can become too much.

I find tracking useful on occasion, and will do it if I really want to focus, perhaps after a busy few weeks when I have let things slip, or if I have a race coming up and I want to be in the best form. What I find much more useful is on a Sunday night (or whenever suits you most) writing a food plan for the week. This gives an indication of what breakfast, lunch and dinners I am going to have and sometimes the snacks I have available. I also include occasions where I might be eating out, or where I am not in control of my food choices like at a conference or if visiting friend. I don't always stick to it religiously, but it helps with shopping, acts as a guide through the week and lets me give my food some thought rather than just seeing what happens and hoping for the best. I do not obsess about this though...life is too short to always know what you are eating for your next meal.

Remember ladies: don't focus on eating well simply to lose weight or drop a dress size, focus on developing a healthy and happy relationship with food and on finding and maintaining the feeling of being in control. Food should never be the enemy; you should never feel like it is a battle.

Drop the diet mentality and find a system that works for you. This will enable you to ultimately be the happier healthier person you want to be. It doesn't have to be as difficult as you may think, just focus on the here and now, taking it meal-by-meal, mouth full by mouthful.

Fitness

The first time I see a jogger smiling, I'll consider it. **Joan Rivers**

People say to me, 'wow with hundreds of races and miles and miles of training runs behind you, oh and lets not forget a business which is all about running, you must absolutely love the sport of running'. Can I let you into a secret?

I BLOODY HATE IT.

The actual running that is.

'Cos it's bleeding hard work. Ultimately I am a little bit lazy and just want an easy life.

I often find myself at the start of yet another race, or heading out into the rain (again) for a long training session thinking to myself "What the hell am I doing this for?" OK hate is a little strong I suppose. But most of the time I can't say that I 100% love the actual sensation of running, and with my cumbersome frame it's probably not the easiest of sports to have chosen. But in many ways I think that is why I like it. I like how challenging it is, and how there are always new goals to be set.

But most importantly, I love lots of other connected things about the sport: the sense of community; the race scene and the social aspects of running as part of a team, virtual or otherwise.

I think what I actually have is a real respect for running as a sport, as I acknowledge the absolute power it has to transform lives and also how much it has taught me about life more generally over the last decade or so.

It is something that adds to my life, in a similar way that dance did as a youngster. That is the trick when it comes to exercise, its about finding something you enjoy so much that it becomes part of your identity, something you would be gutted to have to give up. But that takes time to evolve, and sometimes it's sports or activities that you don't even know you will enjoy that you will end up falling in love with, so the trick is to be open minded and try lots of things. Just like we did as kids. Or was that just me?

As a youngster, I was into dance. But equally I would try anything so found myself trying all kinds of sports: rounder's, football, cricket, gymnastics, swimming, cycling, judo, taekwondo, ice skating... Seriously, I would give anything a go. At secondary school I still had a similar attitude, but things did go downhill a little bit. For a start I wasn't exactly a favourite of the sports department staff (or many of the school staff in fact) and, because I wasn't very talented at any specific sport, the options for me to get involved in things outside of my 2- hour PE lesson were limited.

By the time I left school, I was completely disinterested in sport. Although I was dancing in a street dance group outside of school, which meant at least I was being physically active.

Task 30 - What sport did you play as a kid?

Write a list of all the activities you enjoyed as a child, and then see how many of them you have done as an adult. Why did you stop doing them?

Things seem to be quite different these days for young people, girls especially, and the engagement of girls in sport and physical activity is a huge concern for those working in the health and sports sector.

A school sport review in 2012 revealed that only 15% of girls aged 17 – 18 take part in at least 3 hours of PE and school sport each week compared to 68% of girls aged 10-14, so something is happening during that time. Maybe it's boys, maybe it's peer pressure, or maybe it is something else all together.

Whatever the worrying reasons for these shocking stats, it's clear that these issues are taken with us into adulthood leading to difficult relationship with sport and physical activity. A survey lead by Dove soap found out that over 60% of girls avoid some activities because they feel bad about their looks. 19% won't join a team or club and 15% won't go to school at all, and 13% won't give their opinion in class. This shocking level of disengagement has to be addressed, and I think adult women have to take the lead by sorting out their issues and being positive role models when it comes to being more physically active.

Let's not avoid the issue here. Last year I gave evidence at the All Party Parliamentary Commission on Physical Activity, which was basically a number of members of parliament feeding back on key policy findings and recommendations to increase physical activity in the UK. I spoke about how I had managed to get inactive women active, and the fears that we often have to over come before we can feel comfortable and confident enough to give sport a second chance.

The report was clear in its findings, stating that a lack of physical activity is a habit laid down in childhood – and with inactivity being responsible for one in five premature deaths this isn't something we can afford to ignore.

So many of us focus on loosing weight for our health, meanwhile a whole heap of slim people sit there in perfect ignorance thinking their slim bodies make them exempt from the need to be active every day. Being overweight does not necessarily mean you are unhealthy, and being slim does not automatically imply good health. We all need to be active, regardless of what size jeans we wear, and irrespective of the state of our diets.

At the start of 2015, and possibly capitalizing on the seasonality of New Year's resolutions that come after the Xmas period, a nationwide TV ad campaign was launched featuring a soundtrack from hip hop artist Missy Elliot and showcasing a whole range of sweaty, wobbly, glowing bodies of all shapes and sizes enjoying sport. The This Girl Can campaign led by Sport England was ground-breaking for a government led awareness driving campaign and caused a massive stir in the UK and further afield, capitalising on social media and our culture of sharing, liking and engaging in cross platform digital and non digital content. In other words, the women of This Girl Can were everywhere, and all of a sudden women who hadn't played any sport in years were thinking that perhaps they could, responding not only by playing sport themselves but promoting it to their peers using the ThisGirlCan hash tag.

This media campaign was a direct result of a huge piece of research led by Sport England to find out why 2 million fewer women played sport than men. Sport England CEO Jennie Price, said: "The figures on participation are crystal clear. There is a significant gender gap, with two million more men than women exercising or playing sport regularly. I believe we can tackle this gap, because our research shows that 75% of women would like to do more"

I know that is true because otherwise I wouldn't get 30,000 visitors to my blog each month, and have a community of thousands of overweight or inactive women telling me they want to be more physically active.

It is not enough for sports organisations to put on activities for women and just hope they come - they need to look at the motivations and barriers of women. Aside from some of the normal logistical issues, like time and cost, one of the strongest and most telling themes was the fear of judgement. Worries about being judged for being the wrong size or having bits that wobble came up time and again. Not being fit enough or fast enough to start, or stressing about not having the skills or knowing the rules to give new sports a go.

We are all feeling these fears, we are not alone...we are worried about what other people think of us, just as they are worrying what we think of them. It's ludicrous.

Task 31 – So what exactly are you scared of?
Write a list of all the fearful thoughts you have about playing specific sports? Then tackle each item on your list and ask yourself where that fear has come from, what it's about at it core, and what would be the worst possible outcome if you ignored the fear and did it anyway.

So I faced my fears and went from someone who couldn't run to finding myself with a place for a marathon. Yep. 26.2 miles is a scary old thing to tackle. But actually I have other fears too. There are a number of sports I would like to try that scare the hell out of me...bikram yoga, pole dancing, rugby, snowboarding.

Talking of winter sports, a few years back a good friend asked if I wanted to go skiing with her in Finland. She was visiting her Finnish grandparents. I agreed, even though I had never skied before and Natalie had been skiing from the age of about 3. What I didn't realise until we arrived was the resort we would be taking to the slopes on was where the Finnish skit team train with no beginner slope. Was I scared? Hell yeah. Did I go to the top of the mountain? Yep. I sure did. The young Finnish instructor we had hired to show me the ropes was great, helping me to build in confidence; she failed to remember one important thing though: how to stop! Her exact words, as I headed down the mountain at speed, were, "now we have a problem"

I look back at these moments and realise that nothing is insurmountable, if you have the right attitude and remember WHY you are doing it. The benefits have to outweigh the fear, and it normally does especially if it leads to increased activity over the longer term.

Have you ever thought about how inactive we are compared to the generations before us? Our bodies do not behave like they would have done hundreds of years ago and that must be confusing for our bodies. I never was any good at science at school so my understanding of how the body functions on a molecular basis is very sketchy. However, last year I was lucky enough to see a presentation form Dr William Bird about the impact of inactivity on public health.

Dr Bird is a leading expert on inactivity and a practicing GP, and in his talk he said the words I was desperate to hear a medical professional utter, "You can be fit and fat". (I think I actually fell in love with that man there and then.) He went on to explain, in a very simple way, that although obesity clearly does have an impact on health outcomes for some people, inactivity is in fact the thing which causes the NHS so many problems, and that a simple commitment to moving more often and more frequently could in fact impact positively on many of the diseases troubling us in the modern world.

As part of his presentation Dr William Bird introduced me to these neat little things in our body called Telomeres. Let me explain in the way I understand this now, although the doctor may have a more technical way of explaining this. I promise you this is the only bit of science you will find in this book, so please do bear with me as it makes a very valid point.

So you know how our bodies are made up of cells, right? And that those cells contain DNA, and within that are our chromosomes? Still with me? Well our chromosomes are X shaped, and at the end of each bit of the X are these things called Telomeres that are basically there to prevent the bits of the chromosome from shortening. Now chromosomes do shorten but over a long period of time, lets say 70 or 80 years, or the average life expectancy...they shouldn't be shortening any quicker than that really, but they are. Our poor diets, and lack of exercise are basically wrecking our telomeres and, in a nut shell, our cells are wasting away, confused by our lack of movement, thinking perhaps that we are closer to death than we actually mean to be. The shortening of these telomeres are leading to all sorts of life threatening or life debilitating disease, like certain cancers, heart disease, diabetes, high blood pressure, dementia...and the crazy thing is just by moving more we could put a stop to some of this.

Task 32 – How much more physically active can you be?
Write a list of 100 small things which you could introduce into your life on a daily basis, remember we are not specifically talking sport here we are simply talking about movement or physical activity, so some of this may be household chores, walking to work, taking the stairs at work.

Being more active as a woman is more important than ever, especially in terms of being role models for younger girls. Sport England, off the back of their insight work, came up with a policy document called "Go where women are" to help sports providers better understand this market. Here are the key principles:

1. **Change the offer to suit the women you are targeting -** don't expect women to change to fit sport and exercise. The current offer doesn't appeal or appear to be relevant for many women who would like to be active. Listen to what your audience care about and tailor the activity, marketing and customer experience to deliver what they want.

2. **Don't just talk about 'sport'** – for many women, sport has baggage. The word 'sport' and its traditional image can trigger negative associations for many women. Address this by considering how you present the experience women will have.

3. **Differentiate sport and exercise from other interests by promoting (not preaching) the additional benefits** – sell

what your audience is asking for. In addition to health benefits, which many women do already recognise, sport and exercise can provide the opportunity to socialise, develop skills and spend time with the family. Makes sure your activity promotes these benefits that many women prioritise other activities for.

4. **Seeing is believing.** Making sport the 'norm' for women relies on local women of all ages, sizes and faiths not only becoming active but celebrating it and encouraging others to join in. Relatable women and girls visibly enjoying being active, at their own pace and somewhere local feels more attainable. Take activity into the community and attract new people by becoming part of their everyday sphere rather than waiting for them to join yours.

5. **Use positivity and encouragement to drive action** – stimulating action through fear of consequences will have little traction. Reassure the women and girls you are targeting that they are in safe and understanding hands. Don't let women beat themselves up about what they do or don't have.

6. **Make it easy for women to act** - right time, right place, right welcome, right company, right gear. Address both practical and emotional barriers together to ensure that neither outweighs the motivation to be active. A more convenient crèche facility may only attract those who feel confident with the activity or in a sporting environment already.

7. **People make or break the experience** – ensure your audience are appropriately supported along the way. Invest in the people that shape the experience of sport and exercise the women you are targeting have. Ensure your audience are welcomed, feel cared for and are regularly

communicated with - whether they are familiar faces, new
or have recently stopped attending

As you can see from this list, getting the nation more active needs
to be a collaborative effort. We all have a role to play in this not just
gyms, sports bodies or local council sports department. Who knows
who might be inspired by your efforts once you have faced your
fears? Your kids? Your friends? Your neighbours? Your work
colleagues? This is the action that government agencies need to
happen, action that gets people moving causing a ripple effect that
changes the sedentary culture of this country.

Public Health England exists to protect and improve the nation's
health and wellbeing, and reduce health inequalities. It does this
through advocacy, partnerships, world-class science, knowledge
and intelligence, and the delivery of specialist public health services.
It also writes policy documents, which are there to be implemented
on the ground. The last one being Everybody Active Everyday,
published in 2014 and which opens with a shocking number of
facts,

*Around one in two women and a third of men in England are
damaging their health through a lack of physical activity. This is
unsustainable and costing the UK an estimated £7.4bn a year.*

*If current trends continue, the increasing costs of health and social
care will destabilise public services and take a toll on quality of life
for individuals and communities.*

*Over one in four women and one in five men do less than 30 minutes
of physical activity a week, so are classified as 'inactive'.*

*Physical inactivity is the fourth largest cause of disease and
disability in the UK.*

So surely the simple concept of being active each and every day is a no brainer if you want to live a happy, healthy and sustained life. Regardless of what size you are, whether you are good at sport, enjoy it, find it easy to find time or whatever, you just need to find a way. Right? And remember Dr William Bird said,

You can be fit and fat.

A study snappily entitled "The European Prospective Investigation into Cancer and Nutrition" which looked at the health of over 334,000 people over 12 years suggests that your activity levels are more important than what you look like, i.e. if you are overweight. By far the biggest reduction in health risk was to be achieved by simply increasing activity levels. Moving yourself from the "inactive" to "moderately active" category reduced the risk of death by anything up to 30 per cent. 30%!!!!!! According to the study, "having a sedentary lifestyle is twice as dangerous to your health as being obese."

The government's current advice for adults is as follows

1. Adults should aim to be active daily. Over a week, activity should add up to at least 150 minutes (2½ hours) of moderate intensity activity in bouts of ten minutes or more – one way to approach this is to do 30 minutes on at least five days a week.

2. Alternatively, comparable benefits can be achieved through 75 minutes of vigorous intensity activity spread across the week or a combination of moderate and vigorous intensity activity.

3. Adults should also undertake physical activity to improve muscle strength on at least two days a week.

4. All adults should minimise the amount of time spent being sedentary (sitting) for extended periods.

This may all seem a little daunting if you are going from scratch, so a good starting point is achieving 3 lots of 30 minutes each week. We all have an hour and a half each week, right?

Task 33 – Create a 3 x 30 chart
Being active is not just something you need to do, but whoever lives in your home should be meeting your 3 times 30 allocation of exercise, or more if you can manage it. So make it fun and draw up a chart and plan your activity as a family.

Think about how different the dynamic of your family could be with more exercise, how your life would feel, what your relationships would be like. The trick is to find a sport or activity that absolutely adds value to your life; it shouldn't feel like a chore or something you force yourself to do. It should be a joyous activity (or collection of activities) that makes you look forward to taking part in it each week.

Task 34 – Try a new sport
Write a list of at least 10 sports that you would like to try. Think outside the box. Do some research. Don't let your fears get in the way. Tell other people you know that you would like to give some new sports activities a go and see if you can find someone else willing to give it a go too. Pole Dancing or Nordic Walking anyone?

If you are struggling for motivation, check out www.thisgirlcan.co.uk for an overview of a real range of sports and activities. But also check out what is going on in your location, and what your friends and colleagues are doing in their spare time too.

Task 35 – Set yourself a movement/sports based Big Fat Goal

Review your big fat goal from the start of this book. Is it still what you want to do? Is the scale of it right? Is it challenging enough? And is it going to help you achieve balance in terms of the physical activity agenda?

But where you would find time for this massive goal? My suggestion is to start with cutting back on your screen time, TV, Netflicks, Box Sets, DVDs, YouTube, and Facebook, whatever it is your eyes fixate on while you are sitting on your backside.

A few years ago my TV broke, well it stopped picking up a signal from the outside aerial of my apartment block, so for 3 months we had no TV at all. It drove my partner mad, and he used my mac to stream content like his life depended on it. I was glad of the peace and quiet so stalled on getting the engineer out to fix the problem. My TV consumption after that point was never the same.

Task 35 – Have a TV free week
Do you watch TV when you are on holiday? Or what about when a family drama takes place? So how about trying a week of no TV? Think about replacing this normal family time with something else, something physical. When your week is over, think about what TV you really missed, and which programmes you could happily do without. In the future perhaps schedule TV free days, and keep up some of the new activities you replaced it with.

That should be enough to get you started. But just one final thought. You will see the benefits of increased activity and the taking up of a new sport straight away. You may lose weight, you may automatically want to start adjusting your diet, and your mood and energy levels will have an almost immediate boost. However, your body adapts quickly and if you don't keep challenging it, it will get complacent and those benefits may cease.

This is where you need to be mindful of intensity. Long, slow, sustained activity is great for building strength and endurance, and indeed confidence, but get yourself out of your comfort zone from time to time. Up the speed, push yourself harder, try something new. This is where the adventure is; this is when your body is going to feel alive.

Understand where it is you want to go. Then picture yourself there. If you can picture yourself there, then you can be there. Bottom line.
Cyndi Lauper, Pop Star

Fun

When is the last time you laughed. I mean really laughed. I mean laughed so much that you wet yourself, or fell off a chair, or spat your drink out through your nostrils. When is the last time you had such an enjoyable day that you simply glowed with feelings of abundance and joy.

Charlie Chaplin said "A day without laughter is a day wasted" and boy was he right. But as adults we sometimes forget that, and we now have to schedule activities to remind ourselves that we know how to have fun. As kids of course it was so much easier, fun came to us without us even having to try, we could make things fun without hardly any effort at all...then the teenage years fell upon us and we were told to walk in corridors, stand up straight, stop fidgeting, be quiet...basically to grow up.

But what if you didn't want to grow up?

Sport is one of the few activities that encourage that childlike sense of fun way into our 70s or 80s, if our bodies allow. Yet, for girls we limit our experiences of sport, and therefore fun because during our teens we start getting super self conscious about our bodies. Doing anything we can to prevent being looked at, stopping the inevitable bounce, and getting hot and sweaty.

Task 36 – Can you remember the last time you felt childlike within your body?
Think back to the last time you were completely free with your body, when you didn't give a shit how it moved, if you might fart, pee or fall over...or what anyone else thought of it.

I can remember the last time I truly felt free with my body. I was 13 years of age. I was on holiday in a caravan in Clacton upon Sea with my mum and my 5 siblings. Mum had just sent my sister Jennie and I down the shop to get cake and custard to have after dinner, we decided to race through the caravans to see who could get there first. We were running at full pelt, our faces were red, we were laughing uncontrollably...and then it happened, that moment when you are running faster than your legs can cope with and I found myself flying through the air, hands reaching out in front of my face with a look of shock horror on my face.

I learnt two important lessons that day, one that no dessert is ever worth running for and two never wear white leggings in the vicinity of grass. I have done neither since on grass or otherwise.

After that moment mainly due to the fact that my sister took the micky out of me I curbed my enthusiasm when it come to running, I became uber aware of my body and I never quite got over the embarrassment of skidding on my knees in front of a whole heap of holiday makers. My sister Jennie calls it my "Praising the Lord" moment, as I did look like I was kneeling down to pray.

We still laugh about it now. In fact we created a whole game based on this one incident.

So I have 5 siblings, 2 brothers and 3 sisters, but Jennie is the one closest to me in age. We shared a bedroom and we have since shared a whole heap of experiences, many of which I can't admit to in a book. But lets put it this way; we have had some fun in our times. In fact we call ourselves the "sisters of stupid ness" amongst other things. Some time last year, we were both feeling a bit glum about one thing or another and via text one night I sent her a string of texts that went a little bit like this.

Me   Hey Jen? Wanna play a game?

Jen   Go on then

Me   List the ten funniest things that ever happened

Jen   What like the time you praised the lord? (I knew that one was coming)

Me   lol

Jen   And the time you fell over outside Bagleys (had forgotten about that one)

Me   Soooooo embarrassing, I rocked like a bleedin weeble

Jen   Oh and when you fell asleep on that packed bus on the way home from Carnival that time and the bus doors kept slamming you in your face at every stop. Ha ha

Me   Not funny, but funny ha ha

Jen   Oh and remember when I broke the toilet seat in Aiya Napa and looked like I was skiing?

Me   the same night you were sick in the main square? (Her not me!!!)

Let me tell you, the evening went on like this for hours with text upon text of really funny things, many of which were not funny at the time. We laughed and we laughed. We laughed until we were both crying. When my partner came home he thought something was wrong with me as I was laughing and tears were streaming down my face, I couldn't even explain why I was laughing and inevitably he couldn't do anything other that join in too.

Because that's the thing about laughter, it's infectious.

Who remembers the scene from the film Mary Poppins where the laughter, and rounds of the song "we love to laugh, ha, ha, ha, ha" become so catching that everyone joined in and ended up having a tea party on the ceiling? But as soon as the laughter stopped, everyone came back down to earth with a bump.

Well our "Funny Stories" game was a bit like the bit on the ceiling, the endorphins, the buzz and the connection between two sisters purely reminiscing on our childhood memories was incredible. And we still talk about that evening, as much needed therapy.

Today was good. Today was fun. Tomorrow is another one. **Dr Seuss**

What do we have if we don't have the ability to look back at our lives and laugh? In fact the ability to see the humour in bad situations, as close as they occur, the better. We all face obstacles in life and we all make mistakes where we wish the ground would swallow us up. Forgiving yourself and others is crucial, and being able to laugh things off is likely to help you live a happier more fulfilling life.

My blog has seriously helped me acquire this skill. It all started after coming dead last in a race (that was dead funny), there was also the occasion when some snotty nose kid shouted out "run fatty run" while I was taking part in a race. But the moment that really took the biscuit took place shortly after having my daughter Rose.

Picture the scene. It's 8.15am the alarm goes off, I creep out of bed trying not to wake my 11-week-old baby and my snoring fiancé. I put on my running gear, set my iPod to shuffle and head out into the bright sunshine.

I was running at quite a slow (but steady) pace, but even still I thought I would make it more than 300 meters from my front door. But for once it wasn't my lack of fitness or my lack of motivation that interrupted my planned 5k, it was 4 lads in skinny jeans who clearly hadn't made it home yet from the night before.

The moment I saw them I knew there would be trouble, but I kept going put my head down, didn't make eye contact and I was secretly quite glad that my IPod would be drowning out their hurtful comments... what I wasn't expecting though was the firm slap to my right buttock which I sustained as I passed them.

The little bugger slapped my arse!!!

That was it...the headphones come out and I swore profusely at the culprit, "so you think you're funny?" the guy in question was in his twenties at a guess, of medium build in grey slim fit trousers, trainers and a light brown hoodie...a description I took great pleasure in relaying to the 999 operator.

The boys had walked off round the corner by this point, one of the lads apologised and begged me not to call the police, but the group headed quite swiftly towards the DLR station disappearing before the old bill arrived.

I knew they were long gone, but driving around in the back seat of the police car looking for the suspect was quite exciting. The 2 coppers probably had a right old laugh at my expense, but they were very professional in front of me at least. A report will be filed and CCTV footage will be reviewed.

I could almost imagine the conversation down the station.

Officer 1   So what was your shout earlier?

Officer 2   Domestic violence incident with perpetrator known to be involved in firearms, and you??

Officer 1   Fat bird who got her bum slapped while out running

It is actually quite funny when you think about it. I knew they would never catch the guy, but it's the principle of it. It was hard enough for me to motivate myself to get up and run at that point.

Comments, sniggers and funny looks are one thing, but physical humiliation that's taking it to a whole new level.

But as I said to my sister when relaying the story, I usually like to know the name of the men slapping my arse, or at least hope they hang around after the event for some cuddles.

You may think I am making light of this kind of behaviour, and its not that I am condoning it. Being heckled. Being sexually assaulted. Being harassed. None of these are right, and often they make us feel really shit about ourselves at the time. But ultimately nobody can make us feel bad unless we give them permission.

Task 37 - Laugh it off
Think about an experience you have that was difficult or challenging, was there anything remotely funny about what happened? Can you reframe the event to find humour by narrating it, or imagining things happening in a slightly different way?

Laughter and fun are proven to be an effective antidote to stress and the illumination or even reduction of stress can have an incredible impact on both our physical and our mental health.

Many of us have experienced stressful times where we neglect our bodies needs, and our healthy habits go out the window. We tend to think of this as a temporary measure, and tell ourselves we will jump back on the healthy train as soon as the stress and overwhelm has passed. However, when is life not stressful? And surely it would be better to find a way of managing these difficult times without eating your emotions, or self medicating with food.

The hormone cortisol has long been termed "the stress hormone" as it is released during times of stress to help with pain, energy levels and increased immunity when things are tough. But the problem is when the cortisone hangs around in high levels in the body for longer than necessary that can lead to weight gain because of the production of insulin and an increase in appetite. So stress really can make you eat more, it's not just a psychological thing.

Cortisone is a complex and important type of hormone though with multiple functions, from regulating blood pressure, to the maintenance of blood sugar levels, and looking after your immune system. Finding ways to control this is key though, because over a longer period of time not only can it put a stop to weight loss, but over extended periods of time can lead to adrenal fatigue leaving you feeling tired, lethargic, run down, overwhelmed, unable to bounce back from minor illnesses and reaching for sugary and salty snacks as a way of coping.

Some suggestions for keeping on top of this, aside from stress reduction include

1. Eating regular meals
2. Eating larger meals earlier in the day
3. Choose natural, unprocessed, seasonal foods where possible
4. Taking regular exercise especially in the mornings
5. Avoid over consumption of caffeine, alcohol and sports drinks
6. Keep hydrated with water, herbal teas an vegetable juices

In the next chapter I will talk to you about my personal experiences of stress and adrenal fatigue. But back to the idea of having fun in everything you do.

Task 38 – What do you currently do for fun?
Write a list of all the activities you do for fun, all the things that make you laugh or which boost your spirit. Are you shocked at how little time you so end on fun activities, or does having fun often revolve around your caring responsibilities so looking after your kids or socialising with your partner. What do you actually do, just for you? What lights your fire? Now double or triple that list and make a conscious effort to laugh every day.

If you can find a sport of activity that pretty much promises fun and laughter as part of the deal, you are onto a winner because then being active won't feel like a chore, and will form part of the fabric of your life rather than being something that has to be slotted in. It's why activities such as Zumba, Line Dancing, Pole Dancing, Mud Runs and Obstacle Course races are so popular, its less about the actual activity and more about the social aspects and the opportunity to have good clean fun (well OK maybe not on the mud runs)

Task 39 – How spontaneous are you?
When is the last time you did something which pushed you outside of your comfort zone? Do you still to activities, places and people you already know so therefore you feel comfortable with, or do you experiment occasionally, perhaps while on holiday with more exciting pursuits?

Why is it that when we are in holiday mode we are more likely to try new activities? Is it because we are relaxed and the activities are part of the holiday so therefore more convenient, or is it because we don't care what people think of us on holiday as much because nobody knows you?

Think about some wacky "holiday like" activities you could do that don't require you being somewhere hot and sunny? How about...

- Climbing
- Abseiling
- Open Water Swimming
- Hiking
- Orienteering
- Water Polo
- Tennis (I only ever attempt tennis on holiday lol)
- Golf

Or how about dancing in the rain? Or running in the rain even?

I can remember clearly a time when during the school holidays if it was raining heavily we would all be in doors looking wishfully out the window knowing we had to wait for the rain to stop so we could go out and play, on the odd occasion we got caught out in the rain it was simply fantastic, splashing and jumping in puddles whilst adults took shelter wherever they could, we would literally dance in the rain till our hair was sopping wet, our lips blue and our fingers numb and crinkly. Being out in the rain was simply the best, and as a runner it can feel equally as invigorating.

Finding the fun in exercise is a state of mind too and can completely transform your attitude to exercise.

When I was a teenager a street dance teacher came into our youth club to form a street dance crew for an upcoming youth festival. I was too shy to get involved and had all kind of body confidence issues, so I sat there week after week watching my friends have fun without me, wishing I hadn't been so stupid. One day 5 of the girls from the group were running late and the dance artist asked if I would stand in just so she could sort out the positioning (we were like 2 weeks away from the show). She started playing the tape (yep not even a CD ha ha, it was the 90s) and was amazed that I knew all the moves. I joined the dance group that evening, and had 2 years of incredible memories of being in that group.

So, are you a yes person or a no person when it comes to new opportunities? Do you refrain from new things in case your body can't cope, or people might laugh? Is it easier to be an observer rather than a participant?

Have you ever read the book *"Yes Man"* by Danny Wallace? Its basically the true story of a man who was sick of his life, of saying no to things so decided to instead say yes to every opportunity that came his way, no matter what it was, regardless of how much trouble he might get himself in to. It is a fascinating read and very funny, and despite the fact the book goes a bit dark and weird towards the end, the concept of challenging yourself and seeing where the universe takes you is an interesting one.

Shortly after reading the book a friend (or more of an acquaintance at the time) said she was going to Columbia to visit her stepbrother and asked if I wanted to go with her. I said YES!! And no this is not a story about naive English girls, drug smuggling and finding yourself locked up abroad. Instead it's a tale of pushing my boundaries and being brave for a change. I had an incredible 3 weeks seeing a part of the world I would never have seen, plus I formed an incredible friendship with a woman that is now one of my closest friends. The following year I went on a week long adventure by myself to the Caribbean over Xmas, where I took up the offer of a local beach boy to accompany me on a morning run. I saw a side of the island that most tourists would never see, and nothing untoward occurred outside the hotel complex either. This is the power of YES.

So...say yes to having more fun this year
Say yes to new activities
Say yes to new foods you haven't tried
Say yes to crazy adventures which scare you a little bit (Ok well a lot)
Say yes to staying up late or visiting new places
And encourage those around you to be more yes than no too

Rest, Relaxation and Recovery

If you want to relax, watch the clouds pass by if you're laying on the grass, or sit in front of the creek; just doing nothing and having those still moments is what really rejuvenates the body. **Miranda Kerr, Australian Model**

Life isn't easy. In fact it can be damn right difficult, sometimes even impossible. But the show must go on, and we must find strategies of coping if we want to get on, thrive and survive. If you are overweight you can often feel like things are even more difficult, with all that physical and emotional weight to carry around and the pressure of being judged or feeling like you should be doing something about your circumstance.

With this in mind, you can often fall into the "good fatty" "bad fatty" way of thinking.

This was a set of hash tags that appeared on social media in response to the idea that it was OK to be fat as long as you were being seen to be doing something about it. In the next chapter we will talk a little bit more about this idea of fat politics, but it is a movement, which has really forced me to think about some of these complex issues.

Blogger Stacey Bias in an awesome post entitles 12 good fatty archetypes describes the concept of Good Fatty being "A fatty who is trying or at least *believes* they should be trying to no longer be a fatty" and the 12 types include

1. The Fat Unicorn
2. The (F)Athlete
3. The Work in Progress
4. The Real Woman
5. The Fat-Lebrity
6. The Mama Hen

7. The Big Man
8. The No Fault Fatty
9. The Dead-Early Fatty
10. The Natural Fatty
11. The Fatshionista
12. The Bad Fatty

Do you identify yourself in any of those descriptions?

You see as a fat person, you are constantly under pressure, often feeling like you are being scrutinised by the people around you, what you eat, and whether you take the stairs...you can't just be fat and be left alone.

At a recent Public Health conference in the morning session the term "Getting people off the sofa" was mentioned like 25 times. What the hell is wrong with our sofas? I'm quite attached to mine actually, it serves me well after a long day and when its time to snuggle up and watch a movie with my daughter. So now us fatties are being encouraged to feel shame for resting our weary bodies on the couch.

Now I am all for getting your blood pumping, pushing your muscles to fatigue and generally having fun through exercise and movement that challenges you, but ultimately your body and your mind has to be able to rest and recover too. Sleep. Downtime. Switching off. Are each as important as getting your food and exercise right in my mind, maybe even more so.

As an athlete you often schedule recovery sessions into your schedule, and despite what you may think these are not always gentle massages or yoga sessions, they can also be regular training sessions but just at a slower pace with less intensity. This gives your body time to repair, as you can't be at it 100% all of the time.

When I talk about recovery with my women, I also talk about emotional recovery, particularly when something shitty has happened that knocks your confidence, or injury, which sets you back for a few weeks. It's as important that we take care of how we are feeling about all this health and fitness stuff too.

I recently delivered an 8-week online programme for overweight women testing my 5weeksto5k programme that was first seen on ITV's this morning. I recruited 65 ladies from across the country and made them fill out a short survey to assess their starting points; the data we collected about these women was astonishing.

66% were inactive
73% could run for less than 60 seconds
6% were completely happy with their bodies
8% were happy with life

And a whopping 50% said they suffered with depression

We all know that being physically active and moving regularly is good for our bodies. But our physical health and mental health are closely linked so frequent activity aside from its connections to fitness, weight loss and muscle tone, can be very beneficial for our mental health and wellbeing too.

But it's a viscous circle because we know activity helps with mental health, according to the mental health charity MIND people with mental health problems are more likely to:

- Have a poor diet
- Smoke or drink too much alcohol
- Be overweight or obese (this can be a side effect of taking medication)

So if you have a mental health problem, the health benefits of becoming more physically active are even more significant.

There is of course a stigma to admitting you have mental health challenges, but the truth is we all have varying mental health levels throughout our lives, and I am sure have all experienced times when we feel sad, low, bored, lacking, energy-less, frustrated, apathetic, angry, lonely, or just a little down. For some of us these feelings are sustained and don't go away even when life improves and it can be hard to accept you have a problem and you need some support.

When I was about to turn 30 I had a string of life changing things happen to me. I broke up with my partner of 5 years, I changed jobs to a role where I worried about being good enough, I bought my first home which left me broke and in debt and my grandfather died. This all happened in the space of about 4 months and I guess I just didn't cope very well.

At first I didn't even acknowledge this string of events had any impact on how I was feeling, and thought I was just a bit tired and run down and needed a holiday, but even after having a three week break I came back and still didn't want to go back to work. At the weekends things were not much better, I either went out and partied hard, or stayed in lonely with nothing to do feeling sorry for myself.

One weekend I reached breaking point, I woke up with a humongous cold sore (this thing was epic) and I couldn't stop crying. I got out of bed and within minutes I was back in bed again. I couldn't eat, I couldn't sleep. I knew something was wrong. So I cycled to my local A&E department because I had no petrol in my car and couldn't face sitting on a bus with anyone staring at my hideous face. It's funny because by the time I got to the hospital I felt a bit better (it must have been the exercise) but I figured I would see a GP about the cold sores. He sensed something was up straight away and I broke down. I couldn't tell him what was actually wrong, I was just very sad, and didn't know why.

I saw a mental health specialist who ensured I didn't have any suicidal thoughts and I was prescribed anti depressants, which came with its own dose of guilt and shame.

I had been having panic attacks at work, and was taking time off sporadically because I wasn't very motivated, but then my doctor signed me of for 3 months with stress. Being at home with nothing to do made things worse and in some ways my health deteriorated and I felt fatigue like I had never encountered before.

Every day I woke up feeling like I had been hit by a bus, or how you feel the day after running a marathon (although I didn't know how that actually felt back then). It was a struggle to do simple things like wash the dishes or prepare a meal. And I was soooo bored, doing nothing but watching daytime TV and reading the occasional book.

I went back to the doctors about the tiredness and they diagnosed me with Chronic Fatigue Syndrome, saying it was possible this is what had caused the depression in the first place because I was under a lot of stress and not taking care of myself properly.

So why am I telling you this? Why am I being so candid about a time in my life when I was at my absolute lowest point?

Because having depression is nothing to be ashamed of.

A quarter of the British population will experience some kind of mental health problem in the course of a year, with mixed anxiety and depression being most common. It affects an estimated 350 million people around the world with fewer than half of those affected receive treatment. In some countries, the figure is fewer than 10% due to barriers of health resources, a lack of healthcare workers and social stigma.

The Mental Health foundation tell us that this is a particular issue for women

- Women are more likely to have been treated for a mental health problem than men (29% compared to 17%). This could be because, when asked, women are more likely to report symptoms of common mental health problems. (Better Or Worse: A Longitudinal Study Of The Mental Health Of Adults In Great Britain, National Statistics, 2003)

- Depression is more common in women than men. 1 in 4 women will require treatment for depression at some time, compared to 1 in 10 men. The reasons for this are unclear, but are thought to be due to both social and biological factors. It has also been suggested that depression in men may have been under diagnosed because they present to their GP with different symptoms. (National Institute For Clinical Excellence, 2003)

- Women are twice as likely to experience anxiety as men. Of people with phobias or OCD, about 60% are female. (The Office for National Statistics Psychiatric Morbidity report, 2001)

We are forever talking about exercise and diet in relation to our physical health, yet when you are feeling depressed none of that even matters, and perhaps mental health and wellbeing has a greater impact on this agenda that it is given credit for.

It is important that you seek professional help if any of this resonates with you. MIND would be a good starting point and of course talking to your own GP. Because sweeping it under the carpet won't solve anything, yet with the right advice and support you can be feeling better in no time. You do have to look after yourself too, and there are things you can try even on your darkest days to improve your mood and outlook.

Task 40 – What can you do right now to be happy?

Sometimes when you find yourself in a place where you all of a sudden feel unhappy you don't always have time to change your whole life, or seek therapy to get to the root cause of this upset. All you want is to feel a little bit better now. So write a post it note with 5 things you can try to change your mood NOW and post it somewhere visible.

My five look like this

- Go outside
- Phone someone who makes me laugh
- Get a hug
- Watch a musical
- Plan something different like a day trip or a holiday

Remember what I said earlier, love is an action not a feeling, so no matter how down on yourself you are you can choose to think differently about your body. One of the best ways of doing this is practicing daily self-care tasks.

As well as being prepared, and having some solutions to the moments when you are feeling low I think you can also take some preventative measures by looking after yourself with small acts of self love or self care each day. Over the years I have gone through spells where I didn't really look after my self, didn't bother getting my hair coloured or cut, didn't bother with my face care routine, or taking time to exercise, or even arrange things with my friends. Sometimes this was because life was busy and stressful and I didn't prioritise it, and then at other times it was because I thought "what's the point? I'm still gonna look crap" But self care is not just about how you look, more importantly its about the relationship you have with yourself.

Task 41 – Practice daily, weekly, monthly and seasonal self-care tasks

Create some regular habits that boost your mental, physical and spiritual health, to you remind you (and those around you) that you are worth taking care of. Something as simple as making your bed each day can improve your mood and productivity and help you feel like you have achieved something

My self-care plan goes a bit like this

Daily – Brush Teeth, Wash/Shower, Brush Hair, Put Clean Underwear On, Eat nutritious food, drink water, take 5 minutes to be grateful for what I have, speak to someone I love, hug my daughter, take my pit stop at 3pm, watch a TV programme I enjoy (30minutes - 1 hour), listen to an audio book/podcast, get some fresh air, brush teeth, cream skin, put on fresh PJs

Weekly – Call mum, watch a full-length movie, buy myself something nice, have an extended call with a friend, schedule some exercise (session with a PT is my new indulgence), wash some clothes, tidy my bedroom, taking time to write, read a book, take a long bath, do my nails, blow dry and straighten my hair, organise an activity or trip with my daughter, having a technology free day/afternoon, cook a new recipe from scratch

Monthly – Sort out my clothes, buy myself something new to wear, visit somewhere new, get a pedicure, reconnect with a friend I haven't seen for a while, eat out somewhere nice, have a day off from work midweek, tackle a big cleaning task (although have a cleaner now)

Seasonal – Do something to mark the season (Halloween party, Xmas carols, Trip to the Beach, Picnic), organise a weekend away (to visit friends, or a race), if funds allow organise a proper holiday, try a new activity, get hair done

You may read this and think, "Isn't this what everyone does?" but you may find that your life recently hasn't allowed for you to prioritise your own wellbeing. When I first had Rose I can remember going for 6 weeks without straightening my hair, I wore the same Jeans all week and was lucky if I managed to have a wash some days...its no wonder I felt a bit crappy after a while. I was taking care of everyone else and not me.

It might be that you manage to do all of the above (and more) no problem in which case, do you appreciate each task and notice how lucky you are, do these activities make your life feel abundant? Well looked after?

Further more, do you know someone else who all of a sudden stops doing all those small things to take care of themselves? How about helping them out? and encouraging them to get back in the routine of self-care and self-love.

Keep yourself busy if you want to avoid depression. For me, inactivity is the enemy.
Matt Lucas

An activity, which I have suggested, a number of times during this book is that of writing daily. I no longer keep a regular diary because I write my blog, but it is something I may come back to for more personal things.

Keeping a journal, which has a focus on feelings around your own health and wellbeing, may even support your weight loss or fitness goals. Julia Cameron, the author of *The Artist's Way,* believes the key to diet success is in thoughts and words, not measurements or numbers.

"For 25 years, as I taught creative unblocking, I had seen that my students would become more lean and more fit as they worked with creativity tools. And so I found myself thinking, 'Oh my God, this is right underneath my nose ... Writing is a weight loss tool," she says.

Her book, *The Writing Diet* has some standard dieting advice, including a recommendation to walk 20 minutes a day and to drink lots of water. But beyond that, she says, as part of your daily self-care routine you should take time in the morning to write down your thoughts and then keep an eating journal throughout the day. Sometimes seeing things in black and white in your own writing can be profound.

Task 42 – Build your support team

Have a think about who you have in your circle of trust. This could be a partner or family or friends. But who else do you trust that has your back? This doesn't just have to be people that offer your support pro bono, it could be paid professionals that add value to your life, and as an athlete (which you are of course) having these people in place is key.

Social isolation is known to increase the odds of premature death by as much as a third, with some experts comparing its impact to those of smoking and obesity. We don't beat people up for choosing to be a loner though do we?

Scientists led by a team at the university of Chicago, discovered that feelings of loneliness could trigger a biochemical vicious circle that leads to even greater isolation with an increase in the fight or flight response, making interaction more difficult and boosting inflammation... a bit like the whole thing with Doctor William Birds telomeres!

I have had moments of real loneliness in my life, especially before I had my daughter and everyone around me seemed to be pairing up and starting families. In many ways sport was my saviour as it got me out socialising with others and giving me a focus. The social aspects of sport are fantastic even if you are an introvert, or even just simply getting outdoors where there is a greater chance of some social interaction. A smile or a wave from a neighbour or even a complete stranger can absolutely make your day.

Task 43 – Self Medicate with the happiness drug

As discussed earlier, many of us have a difficult relationship with exercise, thinking of it as challenging, reward less, embarrassing or even as something we should do to punish ourselves for the way we look or what we have eaten that week.

Remember though, exercise produces one of the most powerful happiness drugs in the world. Endorphins. So when life is getting on top of you, you are stressed, and tired and not feeling at your best going out and doing exercise may be the last thing you fancy, but the after affects of joyful movement during these times is exactly what your body needs.

So, next time you are feeling low, get outside and go for a brisk walk. I defy you not to feel even slightly better upon your return.

Sport, physical activity, movement, dance, they don't have to be high intensity all of the time. You don't always have to be in proper kit. You don't have to have a training plan, or leave the session dripping with sweat. Exercise can be used to aid relaxation or combined with meditation, or the listening to audiobooks.

I couldn't imagine a life without sport or activity in my life, and whenever I am feeling stressed or sad I know what I need to do to drag myself out of that space.

Happiness depends upon ourselves. ***Aristotle***

The pursuit of happiness

When we create peace and harmony and balance in our minds, we will find it in our lives. **Louise L. Hay, writer**

I make no apologies that the last chapter may have taken this book from upbeat and informational to a little bit more sombre and scary as we tacked some pretty deep stuff around depression, but I think it was a point that needed making as so often it is ignored in debates around sport and nutrition for adult women.

I recently delivered a keynote speech for the National Probation service about wellbeing and finding balance when it comes to health. I left the stage buzzing after delivering a fun, energetic presentation full of comedy and anecdotes that the audience of probation officers really seemed to respond to.

The poor lady after me however was from the mental health charity Mind, and had to give a 30-minute overview of the various mental health issues we face and the impact of this on workplace stress for this audience of probation officers. It wasn't an easy gig for her at all going after me, and I actually left the session feeling a little glum. But it had to be said, and in some ways you can't sugar coat it. Even if just one person in that room identified the symptoms and felt less alone, then it was worth it.

The stigma around mental health still exists, so despite being committed to talking about these issues I also think a shift towards pursuing happiness may be more palatable, although equally a bit spiritual and woo woo for the masses.

In the early stages of setting up my business I was asked by business advisors to think about my customers, what their wants and needs are. What it is that causes them pain? And how through your products and services you can address that pain?

Many of the people trying to understand my business assumed it was plain and simple weight loss that I would be offering, because there is an assumption that it is the carrying of excess weight that is the pain point for all overweight women, and of course for some women it is this but for many it is not.

But I knew this was not the only pain point for overweight women, mainly because it wasn't my pain point, well not the most pressing one. You see I didn't care enough about getting to a certain weight, or wearing a certain size pair of jeans to go through the pain of extream dieting or high intensity training. I just wanted to stop the pendulum of being on or off my health regime, and to basically stop feeling so crap about myself. For me the pain point was around finding,

- Acceptance
- Happiness
- Peace
- Balance

When I look at those 4 words, I can almost picture what a life filled with those would look like. I'd say I'm not far off from it right now. It is by no means perfection, it's not the fluffy stuff we see in movies, just my life as it is now, but without the crap and with a whole new more positive perspective. A life where I choose to be happy.

In 2014 I was lucky enough to hear Robert Holden, self help guru and Hay House author of the book "Happiness Now" speak at an event about The Happiness Project, an 8 week programme sponsored by the NHS for a BBC documentary called "Be Happy"

The project had a simple goal to just open up a conversation about what makes us happy, to explore ways of creating more happiness in this world through following your joy. Creating but not searching for happiness, which many of us tend to spend our lives doing with varying levels of success.

Robert says, "Sometimes in order to be happy in the present moment, you have to be willing to give up all hope for a better past"

Searching for happiness is about becoming happy which assumes you are not at the moment, and that you have not yet reached it, like there is a void. To follow your joy is something you feel and do instinctively, Robert calls it your "inner GPS" which sometimes leads us to places we might never thought we would get to, as long as we don't block our own path.

On his website there are a range of really useful resources that will help you to follow your joy instead of searching for happiness, including a fab test which helps you asses your happiness. You can try it here

I did it at the start of writing the book and more recently and saw my scores improve, which is probably a direct result of the gratitude's I do daily, and just generally feeling more balanced with things. My most recent test results came through as follows

76 out of 100 – *this is a healthy score. If you want to take your happiness score to the next level, you need to recognise the difference between chasing after happiness and choosing happiness. Happiness is not outside you, it's not a destination; and it's not about "getting there." When you stop chasing happiness, you allow yourself to be more present, more available and more open. This way you find happiness wherever you are.*

Balance in life doesn't just come to you, its something you have to work on constantly, each and every day. The benefit of striving for balance however, is that it becomes easier and easier to notice when your life is out of alignment the more you listen to the signals.

In my keynote speeches I often sign off with a short statement about authenticity and being your true you. I say something like,

"And finally, whatever you do ladies, do you. I spent 20 years of my life desperately trying not to be fat, when in fact it turns out for me, fat is where its at" which always gets a laugh and lots of nods of recognition.

It was a real light bulb moment when that phrase came to me, and women really respond to it as a message when they hear one of my talks, often leading to a standing ovation and great testimonials.

But through the process of writing this book I have been forced to actually look at this statement again to see if I was and am doing myself a dis-service by putting myself in the "Fat Box" for the sake of my brand, although as I already explained I don't see the word FAT as an insult and I am relatively happy with my lot.

I have lost weight over the years through running, and never ever felt completely happy with how I looked but I also know I have sabotaged my efforts over the last year or so through inconsistent training and going of the rails with my eating frequently. So I have to ask myself am I actually scared of being smaller? Am I afraid of what it might mean to my business, to my relationships, to my life if I was to get to a point where I was no longer overweight.

Who would I be if I wasn't fat? Plus size model and TEDx sensation Liis Windischmann identified this exact issue in her popular talk, "An exploration of identity" when she describes the aftermath of loosing a significant amount of weight after becoming seriously ill and loosing mobility. She said,

"My biggest obstacle not loosing my physical abilities, my biggest obstacle was loosing my identity"

Its funny, people often comment "but your not even that FAT!!" like that is supposed to be a compliment, like there is a scale of what is acceptable and what isn't. The fact remains I have a BMI of 32.9, I am classed as obese.

Now I know that BMI is a stupid measure of health, and I stand by the fact I am physically fit and have no health problems at the moment, but I could be healthier, I could have a lower body fat percentage, and less visceral fat (although that is quite low for someone of my size) and who knows what health issues will arise as I get older, or what might happen if for any reason I was unable to run any more?

These are issues I had been worrying about for some time, and it was why I knew I had to trust that the pursuit of happiness and of balance had to take priority over a pressure to be any specific size.

Luckily the invention of the Internet has made it easier than ever to find women going through the same stuff as you, to find inspirational images or words of encouragement when you need them most, two of the useful movements I have discovered via social media for me in terms of changing my perspective on my size are,

- **Body Confidence** a term, which can often be bounded around a lot, especially in schools and in the mainstream female media, like glossy magazines. It sure as hell wasn't something around when I most needed it (during my teens and early twenties) however, are you confident in your body means many different things to different women. Does it mean confident enough to wear revealing clothes, or confident enough to wear whatever you wish. Or is it not about clothes at all and is more about being comfortable naked, or in your own skin...as it seems to be discussed a lot in terms of our relationships with the opposite sex...oh and of course when the beach season rolls round again.

- **Body Positivity** now this is more about celebrating the diversity of bodies out there regardless of how confident you are in your own skin, and without any pressure to look a certain way. It's more about challenging the concept that only one size is acceptable, or attractive and that we should never judge someone on the basis of his or her size.

Health at Every Size is a less know term which I think has most transformed my thinking, but which at the same time I can't 100% support. I have often tried to paraphrase the thinking behind this movement and been pulled up or told off about getting it wrong, so I have copied this direct from their website so as to be clear about their stance

"The Association for Size Diversity and Health (ASDAH) affirms a holistic definition of health, which cannot be characterized as simply the absence of physical or mental illness, limitation, or disease. Rather, health exists on a continuum that varies with time and circumstance for each individual. Health should be conceived as a resource or capacity available to all regardless of health condition or ability level, and not as an outcome or objective of living. Pursuing health is neither a moral imperative nor an individual obligation, and health status should never be used to judge, oppress, or determine the value of an individual.

The framing for a Health At Every Size (HAES®) approach comes out of discussions among healthcare workers, consumers, and activists who reject both the use of weight, size, or BMI as proxies for health, and the myth that weight is a choice. The HAES model is an approach to both policy and individual decision-making. It addresses broad forces that support health, such as safe and affordable access. It also helps people find sustainable practices that support individual and community well-being. The HAES approach honours the healing power of social connections, evolves in response to the experiences and needs of a diverse community, and grounds itself in a social justice framework.

The Health At Every Size® Principles are:

1. **Weight Inclusivity:** Accept and respect the inherent diversity of body shapes and sizes and reject the idealizing or pathologizing of specific weights.

2. **Health Enhancement:** Support health policies that improve and equalize access to information and services, and personal practices that improve human well-being, including attention to individual physical, economic, social, spiritual, emotional, and other needs.

3. **Respectful Care**: Acknowledge our biases, and work to end weight discrimination, weight stigma, and weight bias. Provide information and services from an understanding that socio-economic status, race, gender, sexual orientation, age, and other identities impact weight stigma, and support environments that address these inequities.

4. **Eating for Well-being:** Promote flexible, individualized eating based on hunger, satiety, nutritional needs, and pleasure, rather than any externally regulated eating plan focused on weight control.

5. **Life-Enhancing Movement:** Support physical activities that allow people of all sizes, abilities, and interests to engage in enjoyable movement, to the degree that they choose.

So much of this works for me, and I can see why the people behind this approach do not bend or twist the rules in terms of their messaging as it could easily be taken over by commercial ventures trying to capitalise on its following, while still peddling the diet philosophy.

From my own personal experience I have benefitted a great deal from embracing a HAES way of thinking, but I personally (although perhaps controversially) do not think this has to be mutually exclusive from having weight loss ambitions. The reality is so many women are desperately unhappy with their weight, not only from an aesthetic perspective, but in terms of mobility, stigma, and how it impacts on their life from day...I believe you can still reject the mainstream diet rhetoric, follow the HAES principles and have ambitions to find your natural weight....which is many cases will mean weight loss.

I have found in the last year or two that the militant protection of some of these movements or schools of thought leave women who are simply exploring these ideas scared to post their views on forums, or seek advice.

The good thing is, these online movements are also moving into the offline world, and there are now a range of practitioners, workshops, meet ups, books and resources that help us to better understand these complex issues and open up debate.

Because of digital technology there are so many ways of expressing or exploring the idea of self-love and acceptance, and you can find all kinds of global movements and campaigns trying to turn things round for women of different sizes. This is so refreshing when so often the strongest narrative around is that Fat is bad, Fat is ugly, Fat is irresponsible.

Author of the Harry Potter series J.K Rowling is quotes as having said,

"Is fat really the worst thing a human being can be? Is fat worse than vindictive, jealous, shallow, vain, boring, evil, or cruel"

But surveys and polls time and time again prove that this is still very much a feeling among women, especially young women. A GoldInc/GoGirls survey revealed that

54% of women would rather be hit by a truck than be fat
67% of women would rather be mean or stupid than fat

And in the Girl Guiding UK, attitudes survey 2012

42% of girls and young women feel that the most negative part about being a female is the pressure to look attractive.

How much energy is being spent world wide on worrying about weight gain, or trying not to be fat for fear of what it might do to your life?

But what if the fact we are thinking about being fat even when we are not fat is the reason that we eventually become fat? Does that make sense?

In the book The Secret, which is all about the law of attraction, author Rhonda Bryne talks about the obsession that women often have around becoming fat, and that it is this "dominant thought" which ultimately makes them fat. Because according to The Secret, every thought, feeling and action sends an electrical impulse to the brain and that electrical impulse is like a flashing message to the universe around what it is you want.

"I don't want to be fat"
"Urgghh I hope I'm not getting fat"
"Oh look at her she's fat"
"If I eat this I will get fat"

The problem is, all the universe hears is the word FAT, so that is what it sends you.

Lisa Nichols in the Secret says you need to have "Unwavering Faith" in what you have asked the universe for. You have to believe that is already yours, as if you had ordered it from a menu.

If you desperately want to be but don't believe you can ever be slimmer, how can you be? Your choices, your ability to care for yourself properly, what you attract from other and basically your whole persona are based on what you think about yourself. If fat is bad for you, fat is where you will stay because of that mindset. If fat is where you truly want to stay, then that is fine for you too, only you can decide what is right for you and your body.

I remember in my twenties having all kind of blockages around being active,

- I would never find the time
- I don't drive
- I can't afford it
- I'd have nobody to do it with
- People would think I was weird
- I'd stand out from everyone else
- I'm not slim enough
- I don't have the right clothes

When I look at that list now, I can tick each and every one of those, but it has taken me a long old time to get there because I found it hard to visualise how my life would look with exercise forming a major part of it, and in many ways I wish I had bit the bullet and done it sooner.

I still have blockages about being slim, but I challenge them now

- **I'd have to buy a whole new wardrobe** (So what I love shopping, and it would help me become more confident in my new role as author and entrepreneur)
- **I wouldn't be able to be the face of my brand** (Yes, I could because I have been big most of my life, I could still talk about the issues I do, besides I am about to start growing the business and other women will become the coaches and face of the brand)
- **People might think I am a show off** (Which people? Why would I care? Don't people think that already?)

- **I might put all the weight back on and then what** (why would I if I find my natural weight through my more balanced lifestyle)

Our lives are filled with fear, fear of failure but equally fear of success, because either way it is the fear of the unknown, the fear of change. But nothing stays the same, and it is better to affect the change than sit on the sidelines waiting for it to happen to you regardless.

Task 44 – Manifest the things you want from life
Visualise the things you want for your body and for your life. Create a vision board. List the qualities and experiences you want. How it will make you feel to be content and happy. Behave like you already have that body already have the lifestyle. Take care of your existing body and take steps towards living your dream.

Sometimes though we are our worst enemies because when things start coming our way we bat them away again and find ourselves sabotaging our efforts. A few years ago I wrote a blog post called "Why Half Marathons Make You FAT" and it was about the fact I had run 8 half marathons in as many months, but my fitness wasn't improving because I was in the "I deserve to eat crap because I've just run a half marathon" mindset, unravelling all of my hard work, and worst still not rewarding it with goodness my body clearly needed.

Task 45 – Stop eating for happiness
Keep a food diary for a few weeks and make a note of all the moments where you use food as a way of rewarding, treating or coping with stressful situations. Did the food you chose fulfil the need? Did it make you happier in the long run, or did it lead to feelings of guilt or shame?

I have realised over the years that the popular fitness industry expression "you can't out train a poor diet" is in fact true, I mean if it wasn't, the amount of miles I have put in over the years would mean I would already be a size 0.

But whether you change your diet or not the fact remains that exercise makes you feel better about yourself, more capable, more resilient and more motivated. As your love for sport improves you gradually start to think of your body as that of an athlete and often your food choices change as a result, but only when you are ready for such change.

We live in a culture where food is very much used to reward. Most celebrations involve high sugar high fat foods, and gifts often come in the form of cakes or sweets. We do it to our kids too. Popping a treat in your kids lunch box is of course done out of love, but why do we feel the need to prove our love in that way? Would a fresh and shiny red apple not display the same sentiment? Or a huge hug, or extra time playing on the floor with them after school?

This is not to say that food shouldn't be enjoyed, but thinking about food upgrades in terms of quality and the science behind a diet crammed with fruit and veg, and unprocessed foods as a way of increasing happiness and wellbeing.

We may not be able to always control our weight, or the efforts we put into achieving balance. Sometimes our schedules do not allow for exercise, and sometimes budgets or circumstance mean our food choices are not how we would like them to be. However, we can always choose to be happy.

Task 46 – Do a 30-day gratitude challenge
For a whole month before you go to bed, list the things you are happy for. Even on days where you feel there is nothing, find something to be grateful for. Notice how this improves your mood

and makes you aware of what you have rather than focussing on what you do not.

Just like love, happiness is not a feeling, it is an action. You can choose to be happy, rather than wait to feel happy. You can choose to think positive thoughts, you can choose to be pleasant and nice to people you meet, you can choose to hold yourself in a confident manor and smile.

In hypnotherapist Paul McKenna's international bestseller "I can make you happy" he backs this theory up,

"Happiness is how the mind and body guide you forward towards what is most rewarding for you. Happiness is not just a pleasurable sensation. When you are on a path that brings you happiness, it will guide you, perhaps in surprising ways, to more happiness"

So think about the habits that create balance, notice the pleasurable sensations, and repeat the process as often as you can. After all Aristole told us,

"We are what we repeatedly do, therefor excellence then is not an act but a habit"

Therefore we must just keep on keeping on, being consistent, being the best versions of our self. Surround yourself with likeminded individuals who will boost you up, rather than hold you back. People who want to see you shine as you are.

Earlier in this book I explained the concept of Big Fat Stupid Goals, but I never really went into any detail about how they make you feel. Standing at the start of a marathon just a year after deciding you would run one, having learnt to run, faced your fears and followed a training plan is a strange feeling. People assume that the nerves must be incredible, but I have always found this time to be one of calm because everything is out of your hands at this point. What will be will be.

Getting out the front door, or getting to the start line of a race they symbolise the same thing to me...winning. As women we are so scared of failing, but with running it is impossible. Each and every run you do gives you a gift, and rarely (if ever) will you regret going out for a run.

The achievement of accomplishing your goals, of any scale is great for your self-esteem. It teaches you things about your self, your capabilities, your strengths and your weaknesses, and of course these skills are always transferable to other areas of your life. But the big race is never the end point; it's always in my mind the exciting beginning of the next adventure. A time to refocus, plan and start over.

When I first put plus sized athlete on my business card it was of course a joke, but taking on that persona over the last 2 years has been the making of me. Athletes eat and train; they don't diet and exercise. They work towards a focused goal which as much about the journey and the lifestyle as it is about the outcome. Athletes, are athletes whether they are on the podium or in the training ground, it is simply who they are.

Task 47 – Take on an athlete mindset
Write the phrase I am an athlete on a piece of paper and post it somewhere significant. Get it engraved on your watch, or tattooed on your feet (ok maybe that's a bit extreme) the point is, the more you remind yourself that the journey is as important as the outcome the happier, the more successful, the more balanced you will feel. It will also give you the permission you may need to take your sporting endeavours seriously and to prioritise your own needs.

Things have changed significantly over the last few years in terms of plus size fitness. When I first started my blog in 2010 it wasn't in mind even a thing? However, social media and recently even mainstream print media and broadcasting has raised the profile of larger ladies in sport.

Every time you play sport in public at the size that you are changing the hearts and minds of everyone around you. You will be inspiring all kinds of people without even knowing it. This is not about before and afters, or shocking transformational pictures, this is about the change that happens as women become leaders in their own families and communities.

I don't think women truly understand the power they have to change the health of the world, simply by doing their thing without shame or embarrassment. There is so much negative noise, so much misleading information, enough to make anyone feel overwhelmed. We may feel like we are insignificant to change anything, but believe you me when you step outside of your comfort zone people sit up and take notice. In a real short time I have gone from an off on overweight recreational runner to leading a global enterprise which inspires hundreds of thousands of women all over the planet. How the hell did that even happen? Was it even the plan?

In 2014 I went on a one-day training course with England Athletics called the Leadership in Running Fitness course or LIRF for short. It was a great practical day which gave us the skills and confidence we needed to lead groups of recreational runners. At the end of the day, after we had all had our practical sessions assessed by the tutors we were informed that we had passed and were encouraged to take it in terms to tell the rest of the group what our plans for the future were. I stood up and said,

"I want to be considered the number 1 global expert on plus size running and inactivity prevention for adult women"

The comment was met with a mixture of nervous laughter, and confused faces. I don't even know where that came from, but it slipped out of my mouth without me really thinking it through. What would happen if it actually came true? What if I achieved that goal?

Sometimes we have to just take a punt at something, think big and go for it. But we also have to take some time to picture what would happen if we reached the success we dream about. Walt Disney said "If you can dream it you can achieve it" and he had a point.

Task 48 - What does success even look like?
Go back to your Big Fat Stupid Goal setting exercise, and then revisit your natural weight task results and take those as a measure of success. Think for a while about how life would be if both of those things happened for you in the next 3-4 years. If you reached all those goals how would it feel? How would your life be different?

Despite the fact the world is getting fatter and more money and time is being spent than ever to prevent this trend, nothing seems to be shifting. Are we fat because we are unhappy or unhappy because we are fat? Has the past few decades of dieting culture and the increase of media awareness simply rendered us incapable of finding a normal weight on the BMI scale, or even a weight where we feel comfortable. Will w ever be happy?

I don't think women want to be slim, I think they want to be happy and for as long as I am alive that will be my focus. Happiness will keep me in better health than fighting tooth and nail to be slim, and it is something I can focus on this very moment, today, tomorrow, this year and next.

Let me ask you this final question about your pursuit of the perfect body? How would you feel if you got to that goal weight or had the body you dream of, why can't you feel like that now?

What is stopping you?

"Happiness can exist only in acceptance", **George Orwell**

Final Thoughts

Phew.

I can't believe I find myself at the end of this extraordinary writing experience.

At the start of 2014 someone asked me what my next book was going to be about. I said (I may well have had a few glasses of wine in my system at the time, and was trying to sound like I knew what I was talking about), "Oh, it's all about New Year's resolutions and why they don't work". "What's it called?" they asked to which I responded, straight off the top of my head (because remember there was no book being planned really), "Oh...working title, New Year, Same You" and then before you knew it my PR team got wind of the idea for my new book and I had committed properly to writing it.

Set your intention (even with alcohol in your system) and the universe conspires to make it happen...well, as long as you don't put too many barriers in your own way that is. I even got the ebook cover designed before I had put a single word on the page...it was a big fat stupid goal if ever I have seen one.

It has been an incredible journey for me getting all of this crazy complex stuff from inside my head in some kind of shape. Cathartic yet challenging, like you wouldn't believe, forcing me to confront my own issues and commit to putting my concrete views down on paper, even if there is a chance that others will disagree with them, or that I might be seen as a hypocrite...because I don't always take my own advice, not 100% of the time.

A recent comment on social media after appearing on Sky News discussing the Sugar Tax didn't help,

"Great, an obese fitness expert who is selling a book, perhaps she should read her own book"

And I do!

But without a doubt, aside from this I truly believe that the words in this book will resonate with the women who read them, and support women across the world to make small but impactful changes and adaptations in their life, or not as the case may be and that's OK too.

However, if I am being completely honest, I think the writing of this book was as much about therapy for me than anything. This is me committing to my own more balanced pursuit of happiness, rather than the constant seeking of perceived perfection that I have been so guilty of in the past.

Who wants perfect anyway?

My mum takes great pleasure in telling me I have been far from the perfect child: having been the most difficult of her six kids to carry during pregnancy; give birth to and also then to raise into adulthood, with my peak of disobedience occurring in my teens leading her to absolute despair at times I am sure.

On the 5th of June 1978, when I was placed into her weary arms, the midwife said to her, "You have a beautiful baby girl, with all 5 fingers and 5 toes." Followed by a short pause and then an awkward glance at the doctor, and then the words, "but unfortunately she does have a small birthmark on her left leg, but other than that she is perfect." Finishing off in the most chirpiest of ways realising their faux pas.

That small brown mark originally the size and shape of a kidney bean earmarked me almost from the moment that I was born as being slightly different from everyone else. Unsurprisingly, the small mark grew as I did. Now, as an adult, it stands at almost 6 centimetres long and being the colour of dark chocolate is kind of noticeable on my otherwise quite pale yet shapely runners legs, often leading to people saying "oooohhh what happened" or "ouch that looks sore" baffling me in the split second before I realise what the hell they are talking about.

Task 49 – Ask your parents about what you were like when you were little. Ask them about the specifics. Look at pictures together. Find out the details of your birth. The first few months and the joy you brought to your family.

I sometimes wonder if those early message of imperfection did me any level of damage psychologically, or whether instead it prepared me for what was to come. After being teased about my unusual birthmark at school, I can remember being taken along to my GP while my mum enquired about me having it removed, and being told if I really didn't like it I could consider covering it with make up. I never bothered, why should I, it was part of me and somehow made me unique…something that any child who grows up in a large family is desperate for in many ways.

The point I am trying to make is, I have never EVER felt perfectly normal.

If it wasn't my birthmark, it was my freckles, I then grew a mole on my face (can't remember when as it just seemed to have appeared one day from nowhere) and then when puberty struck: I became incredibly tall all of a sudden…or as I remember it just BIG and FAT. By the time I reached 13, I had already been on two well know diet regimes, and was super conscious of being seen in my swimming costume…possibly the reason I gave up my beloved dancing school sessions shortly after starting secondary school.

I now realise I was never FAT as a child, looking back at photos I realise I was of average size for my height, and even that wasn't incredibly different from my peers...yet I remember so clearly feeling crap about my body, with very few positive affirmations that this was normal to feel like this and that my body was only one part of who I was, or who I would eventually become.

Task 50 – If a young girl confided in you and opened up about her body confidence issues, what simple advice would you give her. Create your own info graphic, post it note or framed picture and leave it somewhere visible for a few weeks.

Having a daughter of my own makes me feel incredibly responsible for ensuring she doesn't have these insecurities growing up. Therefore, I make conscious efforts to reassure my little girl that she is more than just the body that houses her soul, like the incident recently where she told me "mummy, my legs are big like yours" now remember she is not even 3 yet, and her legs are quite big compared to many of the children her age. I simply replied, "yes, our legs are big because they are strong from all that running and jumping we do" which made her smile before she bounded off to play.

There was a fantastic article on the Huffington Post entitled, "10 things I want my 10 year old daughter to know" by American writer Lindsey Mead. I encourage you to find and read the whole article but I will share just the headlines in the hope that you will consider this, not only for your daughters but as a message for you too, because I don't know about you, but I often still feel like a 10 year old girl inside.

1. **It is not your job to keep the people you love happy.**
2. **Your physical fearlessness is a strength.**
3. **You should never be afraid to share your passions.**
4. **It is okay to disagree with me, and others.**
5. **You are so very beautiful.**
6. **Reading is essential.**
7. **You are not me.**

8. **It is almost never about you.**
9. **There is no single person who can be your everything.**
10. **I am trying my best.**

I seriously did not understood what it was to love until my daughter was born, or perhaps instead it was that I didn't know how to be loved and so a whole heap of stuff just seems to have slotted into place since her arrival. I am still 'work in progress' if ever there has been such a thing, but it's moving in the right direction. That's all any of us can hope for.

My body has done a marvellous job of looking after me thus far, considering what I have put it through. All that binge drinking I got up to my twenties, the numerous accidents I have had over the years, including one this year where I fell backwards down the stairs of a bus landing on my neck and knocking myself unconscious (yeah I know, scary right?) and of course I've put it through literally thousands of miles of running over the last 10 years, with little damage to talk of. So I am clearly over that stage of blaming my body for the state of my life because it has done so much for me. All I can hope for is that my body now forgives me, particularly for my failure to believe in it whole-heartedly.

Final Task – So in light of everything you have read in this book I think it is time you took stock of the past year, and the events which lead up to this point and write one final entry in your journal to bring this particular mission of self discovery to a conclusion. Call it an annual report, an audit if you like, or perhaps it's a love letter or even a Dear John. This is not old you/new you thinking. This is about you and your journey. No blame. No shame. This is about positivity and moving forward.

The writing of this book has given me the space, I so desperately needed, to review what I truly think about these issues (my issues) at this specific point in my life. I am by no means perfect and in fact I celebrate that very fact now, as it has very much been like therapy doing each and every one of these tasks in turn myself, many of which have now become daily habits or tools to get me back into a position of balance when things go tits up.

I know it's corny, but life really is an incredible journey to be had and, please help us God, not just a bloody weight loss journey. We have a wonderful opportunity to explore our true potential without pressure to follow any rules other than those of our making. It is our one big fat chance to respond to the environment we each find ourselves in whilst experimenting with the many (and often changing) aspects of our personalities and sense of being. It's supposed to be challenging. But it's also supposed to be exciting and fun too. And trust me it can be.

Life is not easy for any of us. But what of that? We must have perseverance and above all confidence in ourselves. We must believe that we are gifted for something and that this thing must be attained. **Marie Curie**

None of us know how long we are here, on this planet, or what our true purpose is, the least we can hope for is to do and see a whole heap of interesting things while we can and to touch as many lives in a positive way as we possibly can before we die.

It is not a waiting game; in fact we do not have much time at all to waste. None. So please don't wait for a perfect body, perfect bloke, perfect lifestyle, perfect home or for permission of any sort from anyone to do the things you want to do with your life. Do it now.

Be kind. Be smart. Be happy. Be you.

The Retreat

Join therapist Donna Kenney and me Julie Creffield in May 2016 for a week of fun, food and fitness (in that order) on the beautiful island of Rhodes in a luxury retreat like no other.

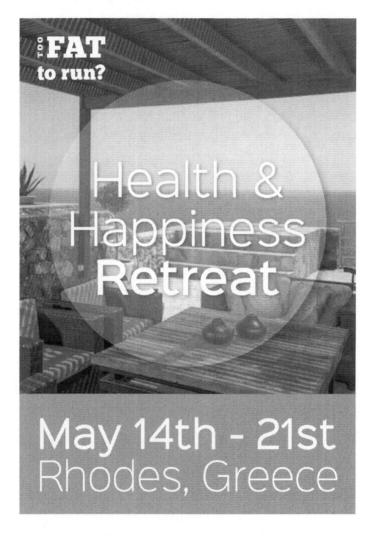

http://www.toofattorun.co.uk/shop

The Clubhouse

If you are looking to join a friendly running club with members from all over the world and of all abilities the clubhouse is for you. Whether you have just started or you are training for a marathon, the training support and camaraderie is second to none, and there's nothing like a virtual kick up the arse to keep you accountable.

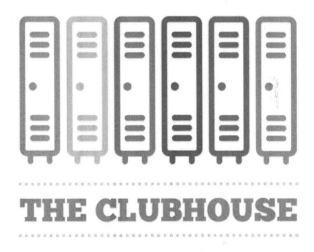

The Clubhouse costs just £10 per month and you sign up via the website **www.toofattorun.co.uk/shop**

I need your help

If you have enjoyed this book and have changed your thinking or behaviour as a result of its content then please help share its message with other women that you love and care about.

Britain's diet industry is worth an estimated £2bm and Americans spend a whopping $40 billion a year on weight-loss books, programs and products most of which we know do not work over the longer term. This is big (and sadly repeat) business, and in many ways bloggers like me with solutions which work and a story to tell about their journey often get overshadowed by the range of new shiny celebrity endorsed diet books we see on the shelves each new year.

There are millions of overweight women across the world desperate for an alternative approach, one which doesn't make them feel crap about themselves, so my task is to get as many women as possible reading this book.

We know that word of mouth and recommendations from people we love and trust are far more powerful than any marketing campaign, so below are some simple ways that you can help other women to find health and happiness.

1. Tell the women closest to you about the book, encourage them to download their own copy.

2. Post something about the book on your social media pages, encouraging women to download a copy

3. Go onto Amazon and leave me a review. The more reviews a book gets the more likely it is people will buy it.

If you would like to share your story about weight loss, fitness, health and happiness then feel free to join our friendly Facebook community for daily inspiration and the chance to share your experiences at www.facebook.com/thefatgirlsguidetorunning

<u>Acknowledgements</u>

As a writer, a coach, or even an entrepreneur (because that is what I am often described as these days) it's easy for people to get confused about who you are and what you actually do, you know the day to day stuff, like how you actually live your life. So let me assure you I am very much a normal person.

I live in a two-bedroom apartment (even that sounds posher than what it is) in the middle of East London; I drop my daughter at nursery 5 days a week, and cook my own dinners and empty my own bins. I don't have a designated office space, I run my global business from an overcrowded desk in the corner of my front room, from an iMac which is on its last legs which freezes at least 3 times a day and I often work with a backdrop of washing up, piles of laundry and stacks and stacks of paperwork.

It's not particularly glamorous, well most of the time its not anyway.

I work alone. I spend hours and hours at my desk trying to make things happen, especially in the early hours of the morning squeezing in the important stuff while I have no real distractions.

The funny thing is I am not at all lonely.

Over the last 10 months or so I have managed to build the most awesome team of loyal, creative and on the most part enthusiastic (when I'm not hounding them to meet deadlines) freelancers picking up specific parts of the workload for me, and it's absolute magic.

For at least the last 2 years I have been doing absolutely everything myself, including packing hundreds of branded t-shirts every week to take to the post office to be sent out, and answering every email or social media message in person.

So I would like to thank the extended TFTR team, and I salute you guys for putting up with me; Marco Media Design who helped me create my website and brand in 2013; Peter who does graphics for me at a drop of a hat; Sharon my eccentric VA who has the patience of a saint; the ladies at Adia PR who I am always threatening to drop (so they push even harder for me and they never disappoint or tell me to do one).

I also have a number of important colleagues where we have a vital, 'I'll scratch your back you scratch mine' arrangement which has been absolutely invaluable to the growth over the last year or so. Vik from VIP digital photography who does all my pictures; Sophie from Fitology who is my new Personal Trainer, and Donna Kenney my therapist (yep I can proudly say I have one of those now...and I clearly needed one).

I simply love you guys.

But the thing which has really blown me away is the amount of in kind support I have been offered from within my community of plus sized women, and in particular my ladies in The Clubhouse.

The Clubhouse is my online running club, which has 160 women from all over the world in it. I am supposed to be supporting them with their running, but in many ways they are supporting me with growing my business, either doing specific tasks like keeping spread sheets of race results, or copy editing my ebooks (yep they have done this too) or helping out at events. My ladies are the most incredible advocates and ambassadors for my venture, and are always there to pick me up when I am low, and give me positive feedback when it's deserved.

It hasn't gone unnoticed ladies and I am incredibly humbled by your generosity.

There have also been a number of special ladies who have gone completely out of their way to drive the growth of this movement; two ladies in particular who work for a well known financial organisation who have taken me under their wing and forced me to be more strategic and ambitious in my thinking. I will never forget how important you have made me feel, and the role that you have played in getting me to this point.

I don't know why I am always so surprised at women's ability to give without the need for anything in return. But I am.

My final thanks of course have to go to my dysfunctional family, and I mean that in the most endearing way. I think I must make their lives quite nerve wracking really, not knowing what I am going to write about or speak about next, what take I am going to have on an insignificant part of our upbringing which I clearly haven't left in the past. They also have to deal with their work friends and colleagues asking about what I am doing next and telling them that they heard me on the radio or saw me on the telly, which I am sure was exciting the first time it happened but a bit like "yeah whatever now".

I love them though...all of em.

And finally to my mum.

I never would have become anything in life if you hadn't have been so hard on me growing up. You frequently reminded me that I was nobody special, in as much as she had 5 other kids to take care of as well as a house to clean and cancer to fight.

I always say I got my strength from my mother, and my running skills from my father (also known as the BASTARD that left us all).

You never explicitly told me well done, or how proud you were when I got my first class degree but rather than have that crush me I simply knew you wanted more from me, and I just got on with pushing myself even harder to succeed and make you proud.

You will never know how much I love and respect you for the way you gave up your life for us and this book is for you and all the women out there just like you that put your life and health on hold to put your kids first...you silly bloody cows.

Thank you to each and every one of my followers, my customers who buy products and services from me and all the running organisations and brands that have supported The Fat Girls Guide to Running to this point.

God I need a drink after that lot.

Here's to world domination and the next 10 years of championing plus size fitness in the pursuit of health and happiness.

Cheers!!!!

14430211R00091

Printed in Great Britain
by Amazon.co.uk, Ltd.,
Marston Gate.